SPORTS AND ATHLETICS PREPARATION, PERFORMANCE, AND PSYCHOLOGY

SPORTS INJURIES

PREVENTION, MANAGEMENT AND RISK FACTORS

Sports and Athletics Preparation, Performance, and Psychology

Additional books in this series can be found on Nova's website under the Series tab.

Additional e-books in this series can be found on Nova's website under the e-book tab.

SPORTS AND ATHLETICS PREPARATION, PERFORMANCE, AND PSYCHOLOGY

SPORTS INJURIES

PREVENTION, MANAGEMENT AND RISK FACTORS

GABRIELLE HOPKINS
EDITOR

nova publishers
New York

Library of Congress Cataloging-in-Publication Data

Sports injuries: prevention, management and risk factors/editor, Gabrielle Hopkins.
pages cm. -- (Sports and athletics preparation, performance, and psychology)
Includes index.
ISBN 978-1-63463-305-5 (hardcover)
1. Sports injuries. 2. Sports injuries--Prevention. I. Hopkins, Gabrielle.
RD97.S694 2014
617.1'027--dc23
2014039716

Published by Nova Science Publishers, Inc. † New York

CONTENTS

Preface **vii**

Chapter 1 Management of Femoroacetabular Impingement in the Athlete **1**
William Postma, M.D., Thomas Sherman, M.D. and Michael Kern, M.D.

Chapter 2 A Summary of Central Nervous System Injuries Associated with the Sport of Ice Hockey **51**
Ozan Toy, Arielle Berkowitz, Ronald Bogdasarian and Mill Etienne

Chapter 3 Protective Headgear for Rugby, Australian Rules Football and Soccer **63**
Con Hrysomallis, Ph.D.

Chapter 4 Predicting and Preventing Sport Injuries: The Role of Stress **87**
Aurelio Olmedilla, Víctor J. Rubio and Enrique Ortega

Chapter 5 Injuries in Hurling and Camogie: A Review of Incidence, Management and Prevention **105**
Edel Marie Quinn

Chapter 6 Resistance Training's Role in the Prevention of Sports Injuries **123**
Ina Shaw, Ph.D. and Brandon S. Shaw, Ph.D.

Chapter 7 Intrinsic Risk Factors That Predispose the Knee Joint to Injury **137**
Terry Jeremy Ellapen, Ph.D.

Index **149**

PREFACE

Consistent physical activity and sport participation is essential for physiological health and mental well-being. Regular physical activity reduces the risk of hypokinetic diseases such as diabetes mellitus, coronary heart disease, osteoporosis and lower back pain. Unfortunately, however, participation in sport and physical activity lends itself to injuries, although it must be stressed that the benefits outweigh the associated maladies. There are many risk factors that predispose the sport enthusiast to injury, and these are classified as either extrinsic or intrinsic. Intrinsic risk factors are person-dependent factors (body mass, skeletal alignment, muscle strength) and rarely cause injuries, but significantly increase the risk of injury. Extrinsic factors include environmental conditions (extreme heat and/or cold, running or playing surface) and sport equipment that predispose people to injury. This book discusses the prevention, management and risk factors of injuries in sports.

Chapter 1 – Hip pain in the athletic population is often a nonspecific complaint and may be due to a variety of etiologies, including: referred lumbar back pain, trochanteric bursitis, athletic pubalgia, musculotendinous pathology, and femoroacetabular impingement (FAI). The lattermost, FAI, is a complex orthopaedic problem, particularly in the young, athletic population, in terms of accurate diagnosis and appropriate treatment. FAI is characterized as painful contact between the femur and acetabulum at the hip joint, often with supraphysiologic motion as required by athletic performances. This painful contact is due to associated patho-anatomic Cam and Pincer lesions on the femur and acetabulum, respectively. Cam lesions are essentially local areas of asphericity on the femoral head, and pincer lesions refer to any number of anatomic abnormalities causing femoral over-coverage. As a result of these patho-anatomic entities and their relationship, the labrum and its adjacent cartilage is subject to abnormal forces and may become "pinched," resulting in immediate pain and likely increased risk for development of arthritis. Diagnosis of FAI is often challenging, as the practitioner must fully elucidate athletes' complaints and completely review pertinent personal and familial medical histories, such as dysplasia, slipped capital epiphysis, Perthes disease, and steroid use to name just a few. Physical examination requires evaluation of the entire back and lower extremity, and familiarity with several examiner maneuvers and induced signs suggestive of impingement is necessary. Selection of proper imaging modalities is paramount, as is expertise in their evaluation, particularly with regards to characterizing the underlying patho-anatomic relationships and understanding the implications and relevance to the athlete's complaints. Much information can be garnered from standard radiographic series, as well as more specific views, such as "Dunn-lateral" and "false-profile" views. Magnetic resonance imaging is also an important modality, and the practitioner must understand its diagnostic role and limitations. Treatment of FAI is evolving quickly and options include: non-operative, symptomatic management, open-based procedures, and arthroscopic-based procedures. Surgical goals are to restore the normal anatomic relationships of the hip and preserve or restore the chondro-labral complex, while appropriately managing expectations. The methods by which this is achieved are quickly expanding and the practitioner involved in the care of athletes, must be able to appropriately counsel the athlete in this regard.

Chapter 2 – *Objective:* To determine the types of injuries affecting the Central Nervous System (CNS) throughout the history of ice hockey and the estimated incidence of each type of CNS injury based on the literature. *Background:* Ice hockey is a contact sport characterized by high acceleration and deceleration forces, fast skating and puck velocities, body checking and forceful stick use. Athletes can receive impacts from opposing players, the boards, pucks, sticks, and goal posts. These aspects of ice hockey pose risks for injury to the brain and spinal cord. Identifying CNS injuries and associated incidence in ice hockey will help clinicians to better inform participating athletes. *Methods:* The authors conducted a literature search via Pubmed. Additionally, they utilized Google and Wikipedia to find media reports regarding CNS injuries in ice hockey. The authors used the following search terms: hockey concussion, hockey second impact syndrome, hockey spinal cord injury, hockey paralysis, hockey head trauma, hockey death. *Results & Conclusion:* The following CNS injuries were the most common: Concussion (0.2 to 6.6 per 1000 player hours) and Spinal Cord Injury (5 per 1000 player hours). Other rare injuries of undetermined incidence include: Second Impact Syndrome, Subarachnoid Hemorrhage, Subdural Hematoma, Epidural Hematoma, Spinal Cord Concussion, and Vertebral Hemorrhage. Controversial associations with long term consequences of head impact in ice hockey include Post-Concussive Syndrome and Chronic Traumatic Encephalopathy (CTE). It is the authors' recommendation that all ice hockey players, their parents, and healthcare professionals are informed of the risks of the game.

Chapter 3 – Rugby, Australian Rules football (ARF) and soccer have high participation rates in numerous countries. A consequence of contact and collision sports is a notable injury rate and of particular concern is head injury, especially concussion. A countermeasure intended to reduce head injury prevalence in these football codes is non-obligatory protective soft-shell headgear. The adoption rate of this type of headgear for rugby (7 to 27%) was found to be higher than for ARF (2 to 8%). The main reason given for not wearing headgear was discomfort. Laboratory studies of soccer headgear demonstrated significant impact attenuation during scenarios simulating head to head contact. Laboratory studies of ARF and rugby headgear have shown that thickness is directly related to impact attenuation and that the type of head form and impact surface greatly influences the test results. Randomised controlled trials with teenage rugby union players did not find headgear significantly reduced concussion rate or other head injuries. There was one attempted randomised controlled trial with ARF but was unable to be completed because of poor compliance with wearing headgear; this is a major challenge for researchers. One retrospective study found that soccer headgear reduced the proportion of concussions for collegiate athletes. There is some evidence as well as inconsistent results from prospective and retrospective studies that headgear may reduce concussion or superficial head injuries in rugby. The weight of the evidence suggests that the headgear assessed so far cannot be relied on its own to significantly reduce concussion rate but should not be dismissed completely.

Chapter 4 – Hardly any sport practitioner would have finished his/her career without suffering at least one sport injury. Sport injury is a broadly spread out morbidity condition sustained as a result of an energy transfer when the specific tissue or organ is no longer able to resist the biomechanical forces that stress it. Traditionally, athlete has been viewed as a mere injury container and the injury itself as a broken piece that should be fixed up. Despite of such outlook, psychological research has shown athletes play an active role on the process of becoming injured and several psychosocial variables might influence on such. According to the seminal Andersen and Williams model, the key psychological factor related to sport injury occurrence is the stress response. The present paper focuses on the preinjury phase, reviewing the concept of stress and analyzing the mechanisms involved in sport injury occurrence. It also reviews the experiences of interventions aimed to cope with stress and the empirical evidence of such interventions preventing sport injuries.

Chapter 5 – *Background:* Hurling, and its female equivalent, camogie, are Irish field sports played with a stick called a hurley and a ball called a sliotar. Both sports have some similarities to field hockey and the Scottish sport of shinty. Hurling is a contact sport and various associated injury patterns have been recognised. Players can use personal protective equipment in the form of helmets, handguards, mouthguards and shinguards. As of 2010, wearing of a helmet with a faceguard is mandatory for all players during both training and match play. *Injury Patterns:* A study of attendances at an Irish emergency department showed that 12.3% of orthopaedic presentations were sports related; in another study 41% of sports related injuries were due to hurling. The most common injuries now encountered are hand injuries, although head injuries are also common. Serious head, facial and eye injuries have been reported and permanent visual deficits have been sustained. Injuries to the external ear, spine, teeth and muscular injuries have also all been described. *Injury Prevention:* It has been shown that head injuries are more common in players not wearing helmets. Introduction of helmets with faceguards has dramatically reduced the incidence of head trauma. Hurling related facial fractures halved over a 20 year period following introduction of voluntary helmet use and a significant reduction in eye injury rates was seen in adolescents following introduction of mandatory helmet wearing. However, current helmet design does not protect the external ear and players are not entirely satisfied with the helmet performance. With reductions in head injury rates, hand injury has become more common. In fact, a recent study has shown an association between helmet wearing and hand injury. The majority of hurling and camogie players have tried using commercially available handguards but <5% of players regularly use them. The majority of hand fractures occur in players not wearing any hand protection. *Conclusions:* In summary, hurling and camogie related trauma is common and can be significant. Use of protective equipment has been shown to reduce head and facial injuries. However, hand trauma remains a significant problem, requiring development of better, more acceptable preventive strategies.

Chapter 6 – It is generally accepted that regular scientifically-designed resistance training programs result in numerous benefits in both competitive and recreational athletes including improvements in muscle strength and power, increases in muscle size all leading to improvements in sports performance. In addition, resistance training has also been suggested to reduce the risk for musculoskeletal injuries or even reduce the severity of such injuries in athletes. In this regard, resistance training can strengthen muscles, bones and connective tissue making them less susceptible to damage and more able to withstand the demands of sport and physical activity. Although studies reporting the direct effect of resistance training on injury rate reduction are limited, the physiological adaptations seen consequent to resistance training on muscles, bones and connective tissue does imply enhanced protection against musculoskeletal injuries. Reducing the incidence of injury by engaging in a resistance training program is as beneficial for the non-competitive beginner as it is for the competitive athlete. Thankfully, many competitive and recreational athletes already perform resistance training as a part of their usual conditioning programs. However, there is an increasing need to engage in resistance exercises that reproduce the performance of the sport and/or motion specific activities. These specific types of resistance exercises should also be performed following the testing of athletes for agonist and antagonist muscle strength imbalances as such data can be utilized to identify athletes with a predisposition for injury. In these cases, resistance training may then be performed to correct the observed imbalance and hopefully reduce the incidence and/or severity of future injury. While evidence suggests that a targeted resistance-based approach can prevent musculoskeletal injuries or even reduce the severity, recent evidence suggests that resistance can also be utilized to accelerate recovery from such injuries and is increasingly being used in this role as an excellent alternative method of rehabilitating sports injuries. However, it must be noted that the improper execution of resistance exercises can themselves be cause for injury, especially in the youth. As such, resistance-focused workouts should be performed with proper form and technique or under the supervision of qualified and certified trainers. In conclusion, despite the old belief of resistance training being ineffective and unsafe, resistance training has been shown to decrease sport injuries and their severity, rehabilitation time relative to non-resistance trained individuals and should be considered as an important component to include in any fitness or sport-performance program, even in the youth due to their ever- lengthening and increasingly earlier competitive careers.

Chapter 7 – The objective of this chapter is to enlighten developing sport medicine practitioners and students on the impact of various intrinsic risk factors that can predispose an athlete to knee pain and injury. Athletes are subjected to both extrinsic (external) and intrinsic (internal) factors that facilitate injury. The pathomechanics of intrinsic factors is not investigated frequently by the sporting fraternity. This chapter reviews the following intrinsic risk factors of knee injury: tibio-femoral alignment in both the sagittal and frontal planes, patella-femoral orientation within the femoral trochlear and the presence of deviant quadriceps, A-angle and torsion angles. The non-invasive clinical techniques that can be used to determine risk of injury and possible soft tissue that has been damaged, will be described. Kendall protocol for lower limb alignment in both the frontal and sagittal planes is used to determine the presence of genu varum (bow leg), genu valgum (knock knees) and genu recurvatum (hyper-extension of the tibio-femoral joint). The presence of the abovementioned clinical conditions is also related to the asymmetrical strength of the surrounding musculature and flaccid ligaments. Prentice's patella orientation techniques are used to identify abnormal patella orientation within femoral trochlear, such as patella alta, baja and medial squinting. The Livingstone and Spaulding technique was used to measure quadriceps angle, while the author uses Prentice's technique to measure the A-angle. Techniques to measure torsion angles are also included.

In: Sports Injuries
Editor: Gabrielle Hopkins
ISBN: 978-1-63463-305-5

Chapter 1

Management of Femoroacetabular Impingement in the Athlete

William Postma, M.D., Thomas Sherman, M.D. and Michael Kern, M.D.
MedStar Georgetown Orthopaedic Institute, Washington, D.C., US

Abstract

Hip pain in the athletic population is often a nonspecific complaint and may be due to a variety of etiologies, including: referred lumbar back pain, trochanteric bursitis, athletic pubalgia, musculotendinous pathology, and femoroacetabular impingement (FAI). The lattermost, FAI, is a complex orthopaedic problem, particularly in the young, athletic population, in terms of accurate diagnosis and appropriate treatment. FAI is characterized as painful contact between the femur and acetabulum at the hip joint, often with supraphysiologic motion as required by athletic performances. This painful contact is due to associated patho-anatomic Cam and Pincer lesions on the femur and acetabulum, respectively. Cam lesions are essentially local areas of asphericity on the femoral head, and pincer lesions refer to any number of anatomic abnormalities causing femoral over-coverage. As a result of these patho-anatomic entities and their relationship, the labrum and its adjacent cartilage is subject to abnormal forces and may become "pinched," resulting in immediate pain and likely increased risk for development of arthritis.

Diagnosis of FAI is often challenging, as the practitioner must fully elucidate athletes' complaints and completely review pertinent personal and familial medical histories, such as dysplasia, slipped capital epiphysis, Perthes disease, and steroid use to name just a few. Physical examination requires evaluation of the entire back and lower extremity, and familiarity with several examiner maneuvers and induced signs suggestive of impingement is necessary. Selection of proper imaging modalities is paramount, as is expertise in their evaluation, particularly with regards to characterizing the underlying patho-anatomic relationships and understanding the implications and relevance to the athlete's complaints. Much information can be garnered from standard radiographic series, as well as more specific views, such as "Dunn-lateral" and "false-profile" views. Magnetic resonance imaging is also an important modality, and the practitioner must understand its diagnostic role and limitations. Treatment of FAI is evolving quickly and options include: non-operative, symptomatic management, open-based procedures, and arthroscopic-based procedures. Surgical goals are to restore the normal anatomic relationships of the hip and preserve or restore the chondro-labral complex, while appropriately managing expectations. The methods by which this is achieved are quickly expanding and the practitioner involved in the care of athletes, must be able to appropriately counsel the athlete in this regard.

INTRODUCTION

Femoroacetabular impingement (FAI) is a condition characterized by altered anatomic morphology of the hip joint that leads to painful and pathologic abutment of the proximal femur and acetabulum. This abnormal contact results in intra-articular pathology including labral and cartilage injury. It is a recognized source of pain and dysfunction, particularly amongst athletes, and a likely precursor to early hip degeneration (Ganz, 2003). FAI is classified into three major categories on the basis of the anatomic deformities present: cam-type, pincer-type, and combined cam and pincer patterns.

A cam-type deformity is defined as an abnormal prominence of the anterosuperior proximal femoral head-neck junction (FIGURE 1). During hip motion, particularly flexion, the cam deformity generates a shear force on the abutting anterolateral acetabulum. Repetitive supraphysiologic hip motion required in certain athletic activities exacerbates this abnormal contact as the prominent cam-deformity is squeezed under the acetabular rim, which may result in significant intra-articular injury, including labral and chondral damage (Leunig, 2005). Typically, this is most severe at the chondrolabral junction on the anterolateral acetabular rim, as the shear force of the abutting femur causes delamination from the underlying subchondral bone; however, labral or chondral injury may also occur in isolation (Beck, 2005; Ito, 2001).

The origin of cam deformities is debated. Slipped capital femoral epiphyses (SCFEs) are a recognized precursor to the development of cam-type deformities, and some hypothesize that subtle or subclinical slips during childhood may lead to cam deformities during adolescence and adulthood (Klit, 2014; Castañeda, 2013; Giles, 2013; Goodman, 1997). Others theorize that increased physical activity during adolescence contributes to abnormal development of the proximal femoral physis that leads to the characteristic and problematic morphology during adolescence and adulthood (Carsen, 2014; Siebenrock, 2013a and 2013b; Ng, 2011). It is also possible that cam deformities represent niduses of reactive bone formation from apposition of the anterosuperior head-neck junction and the acetabulum independent of physeal development. Regardless of their origin, cam deformities are characterized on the basis of their radiologic appearance, of which multiple methods of evaluation have been described and will be discussed in detail.

A pincer-type deformity is characterized as a bony prominence at the anterolateral acetabulum that may result in abnormal contact with the proximal femur (Figure 1). Several aspects of acetabular morphology are relevant to this deformity and include: version, inclination, depth, and localized abnormal bone formation. The resulting prominence may propagate entrapment of the labrum between the acetabular rim and the proximal femur as well as cartilage damage from the shear force generated by squeezing of the deformity into the acetabulum. The presence of a concomitant cam deformity makes this abutment more severe and with repetitive impaction of the femur and acetabulum, synovial herniation through areas of cortical damage may also occur.

Cam-type deformities are more common in males, while pincer-type deformities occur with approximately equal frequency in males and females (Byrd, 2009a & 2009b). In general, cam-type deformities are more clinically relevant during adolescence and young adulthood while pincer-type deformities are more symptomatic during middle adulthood (Byrd, 2009a & 2009b). FAI morphology is more likely to be problematic in the athlete overall, as repetitive supraphysiologic motion of the hip required of these individuals may exacerbate painful abutment and propagate intra-articular pathology. Although this abnormal contact may lead to early degenerative joint disease in the long-term, it also results in painful cartilage and labrum injuries in the short term, which have a significant impact on athletic performance and overall function.

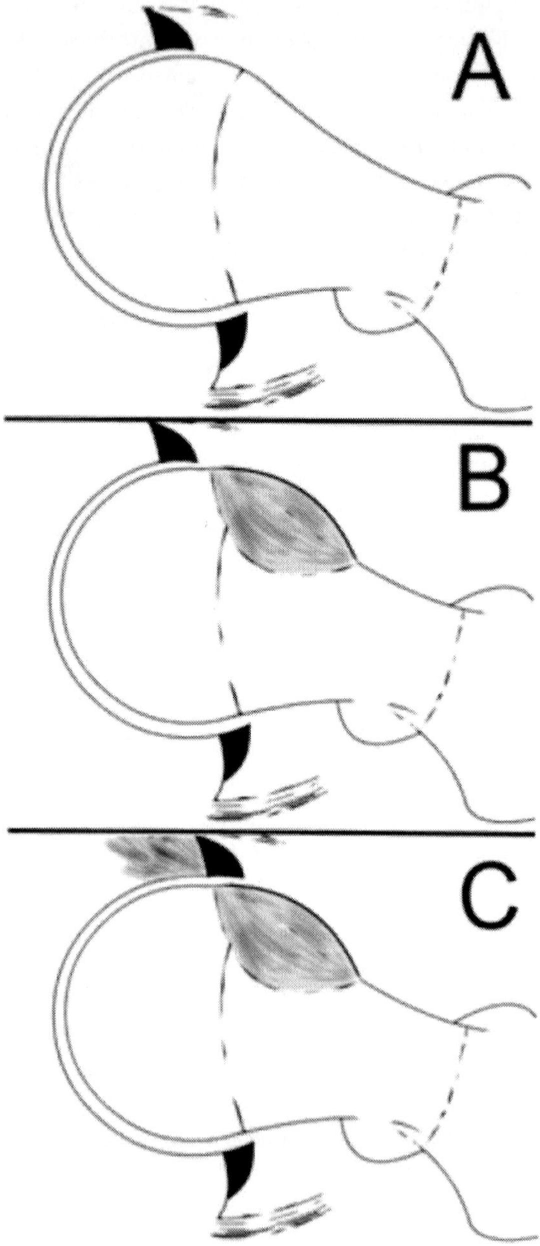

Figure 1. Axial illustrations of the hip. (A) Normal hip anatomy; (B) Cam deformity on the anterior femoral head-neck junction; (C) Cam and pincer deformities.

History of FAI

Abutment of the femoral neck on the acetabular margin was first proposed as a precursor to the development of hip osteoarthritis (OA) by Smith-Petersen in 1936 (Smith-Petersen, 2009). Stulberg and Harris expanded upon this concept in 1974 when they recognized an increased prevalence of pistol-grip deformities described as a loss of the normal concavity on the anterosuperior femoral head-neck junction in patients with early OA. These reports formed a basis for the theory that morphological deformities of both the femur and acetabulum predispose individuals to repetitive intra-articular injury from abnormal contact forces through the joint. However, the modern theory of impingement is credited to Ganz and colleagues from their series that first described impingement as a sequela of other hip conditions in the 1990s. These reports included femoral neck fractures and those that had undergone periacetabular osteotomies for dysplasia (Eijer, 2001; Myers, 1999). Additionally, impingement following SCFE was described around the same time (Rab, 1999).

Patients with these predisposing conditions comprise only a small percentage of those with impingement symptoms. Furthermore, many patients diagnosed with idiopathic hip OA fail to yield a clear pathologic cause. Following their initial reports, Ganz and colleagues (2003) recognized that cam and pincer deformities, which they described as developmental defects, were also significant sources of impingement that ultimately led to OA. They proposed that abutment of FAI morphology was the pathomechanism for the vast majority of idiopathic OA (Ganz, 2003 & 2008). Although interest in FAI initially revolved around its potential relationship to OA, more recently, FAI has also been recognized as a significant source of pain and disability in young individuals (Wenger, 2004; Byrd, 2014). This is especially relevant to athletes, as many of the requisite repetitive and supraphysiologic maneuvers for competition cause forceful abutment of the femur and acetabulum.

Epidemiology

When evaluating patients with FAI, it is important to recognize that radiologic FAI does not necessarily imply symptomatic impingement. Although FAI morphology is characterized on the basis of radiologic appearance, it is a dynamic biomechanical process. In the case of athletes, certain activities and physical maneuvers that would normally be tolerated by a morphologically normal hip cause abutment in individuals with cam and pincer deformities. This potentially leads to painful intra-articular damage. Furthermore, as athletes push their bodies beyond their normal physiologic limits on a repetitive basis, greater forces are transferred through the areas of abnormal contact, which results in acceleration of intra-articular chondrolabral breakdown. Likewise, individuals with cam and pincer lesions who do not regularly perform activities causing forceful impingement may not develop intraarticular damage, pain, or disability.

To this end, several studies have investigated the prevalence of radiologic FAI in the general population. Laborie et al. (2001) performed a radiographic study of 2081 young individuals without symptoms of FAI. Thirty-five percent of males and 10.2% of females had radiologic evidence of cam-type deformities, and pincer-type deformities were identified in 34.3% of males and 16.6% of females. In a separate study of 244 asymptomatic male military recruits, Reichenbach et al. (2010) reported an overall frequency of 24% for cam deformities. The prevalence of radiologic FAI will be discussed in further detail in the "Imaging" section.

The potential link between FAI and the subsequent development of OA has also been investigated in several large radiographic studies. Evaluation of 3000 patients in the Copenhagen Osteoarthritis study by Gosvig et al. (2008) found a prevalence of 17% for cam deformities in males and 4% in females but found no association with radiographic signs of OA. However, other population-based studies do support a relationship between FAI associated deformities and osteoarthritis (Nicholls, 2011). Despite these conflicting results, FAI is typically viewed as a risk factor for the development of OA.

It should be noted that many of these large radiographic studies have several limitations, not the least of which is that FAI morphology is typically evaluated using limited radiographic information (a single AP view of the pelvis, for example). Thus, radiologic FAI may be missed, as multiple radiographic views are often required for adequate characterization. Additionally, evaluation of FAI in older patients can be difficult because radiologic signs of osteoarthritis may be indistinguishable from morphologic features of FAI. These studies provide some insight regarding the relationship of FAI to OA; however, further research is required to fully elucidate this relationship.

EPIDEMIOLOGY OF FAI IN ATHLETES

The association between athletic participation and altered hip morphology was first proposed by Murray and Duncan 1971, as they observed an increased incidence of femoral neck deformities in male athletes. They theorized that these deformities occurred after partial epiphysiolysis in the proximal femur from overloading of the joint. Subsequent studies have supported this hypothesis, also reporting high rates of cam deformities in active young patients.

Radiologic FAI is typically more prevalent in athletes than in the general population. Participation in certain sports is also more strongly associated with the radiologic presence of these deformities than others. For instance, ice hockey and basketball players demonstrate higher rates of FAI morphology than skiers and ballet dancers (Siebenrock, 2013a & 2013b; Duthon, 2013; Kolo, 2013). A high rate of FAI morphology has also been reported in football players. In fact, one study reported that 95% of collegiate football players had at least one radiologic sign of FAI-type morphology (Kapron, 2011). An association between soccer and FAI has been reported as well; however, conflicting reports have resulted in some debate regarding this relationship (Lahner, 2014a; Johnson, 2012). In general, however, athletes with hip pain are more likely to have radiological evidence of FAI than those whom are asymptomatic (Siebenrock, 2013b).

Despite these observations, the relationship of athletic participation and FAI morphology is far from fully defined. It is unclear whether the association between FAI and athletics is one of causation, and the nature of such a potential relationship is debated amongst those that ascribe to this theory. For instance, some contend that FAI morphology is the consequence of general overload from athletic participation, while others believe that it is only certain physical maneuvers unique to some sports that lead to clinically symptomatic FAI. Clearly, additional research is required to fully define this relationship.

PRESENTATION

Patients with FAI typically complain of anterior hip or groin pain. The onset of pain is usually insidious and progressive, although some patients may identify a specific injury as the inciting event. The pain is characteristically worse with activity, and usually exacerbated by flexion and internal rotation of the hip.

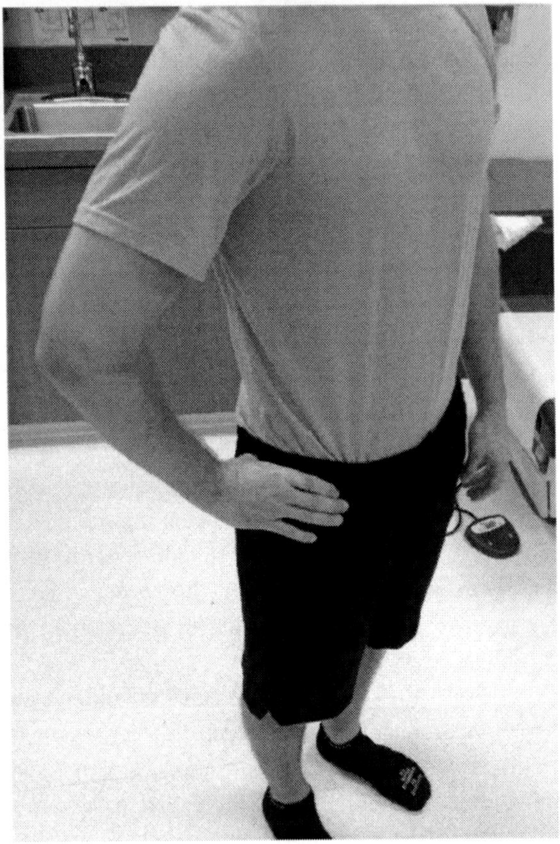

Figure 2. Patient displaying the "c-sign" typical of FAI. The hand is cupped just proximal to the greater trochanter and the fingers gripping the groin.

It is not unusual for patients to note that the extremes of motion are most painful, which likely correlates with the point that the acetabulum and femoral head-neck junction engage causing impingement of intraarticular chondrolabral structures. Patients with intraarticular hip pathology classically describe their pain with the "C-sign", cupping their hand just above the greater trochanter and fingers gripping the groin (Figure 2). Some patients, particularly those with cam deformities, may report decreased hip range of motion. In patients with coexisting intraarticular injuries, mechanical symptoms such as catching, locking, or clicking may be present and triggered by specific movements. Activities that provoke symptoms are typically those that require maximal hip flexion, such as running up stairs, or hip extension against resistance, such as jumping or rising from a squatting position (Clohisy, 2009b). As opposed to those with isolated cam-type deformities, patients with pincer deformities tend to report more severe and/or constant pain. This observation may be explained by the increased incidence of intrasubstance labral tears in these patients and the fact that the labrum has innervation with nociceptive fibers (Kim, 1995).

PHYSICAL EXAM

The classic physical finding found on examination most associated with FAI is limited internal rotation. Although patients with FAI generally have reduced internal rotation compared to the general population and athletes with more severe radiologic FAI have greater restriction of internal rotation, the reliability of this finding is limited by several factors (Clohisy, 2009b; Kapron, 2011). First, there is marked variability in baseline motion amongst individuals. Second, many patients with unilateral impingement symptoms have bilateral FAI morphology. Thus, these individuals may have decreased rotation symmetrically. Finally, although uncommon, some individuals with clinical impingement may actually have increased rotation of the hip.

Examination should begin with inspection, and gait should be observed. A Trendelenberg gait may be found in patients with hip pain secondary to dysplasia; an antalgic gait is nonspecific and may be observed in patients with any intraarticular pathology. The examiner should then proceed with palpation of the involved hip and pelvis region, which may elicit valuable diagnostic information. Tenderness over the greater trochanter may be indicative of trochanteric bursitis. Discomfort over the anterior pubis or pain triggered with resisted "sit-ups" may be representative of athletic pubalgia.

Several provocative examination maneuvers have been described with regards to hip pain in general and FAI in particular. Log-roll of the hip is highly specific for pathology of the hip joint of any cause (Figure 3). Recreation of impingement symptoms may be elicited by the examiner using the anterior impingement test, which passively places the hip in flexion, adduction, and internal rotation (FADIR) (Figure 4). The asymptomatic side should also be examined for comparison, as this may be a painful maneuver even in the absence of FAI. The sensitivity of this test is reported as 88-99% (Philippon, 2007; Clohisy, 2009b).

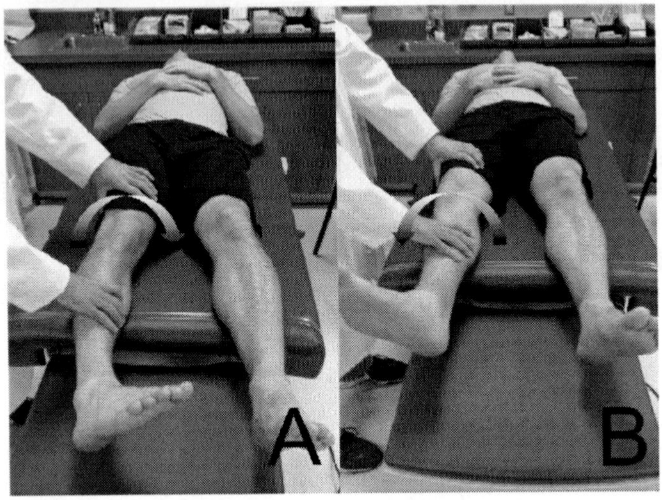

Figure 3. The log-roll test is performed with the patient supine and the extremity is (A) internally and (B) externally rotated at the hip by the examiner. Groin pain is specific for intra-articular hip pathology.

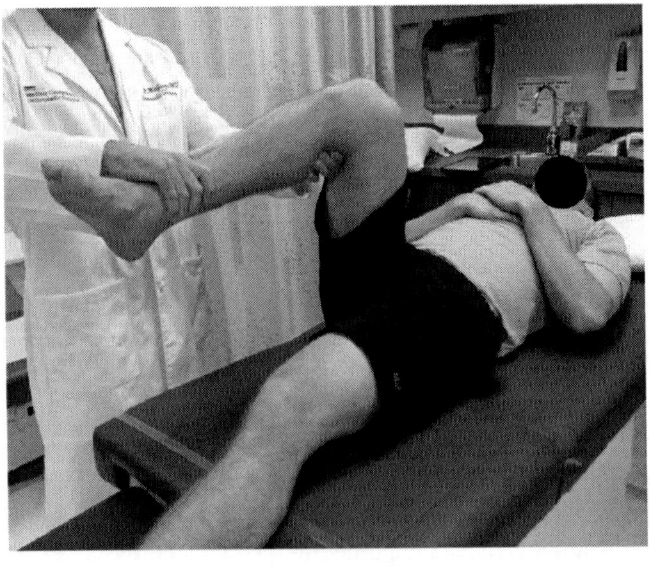

Figure 4. The anterior impingement or FADIR test is performed with the patient supine and examiner on the affected side. The hip is flexed passively to 90° and adducted to approximate the femur and acetabulum. Internal rotation then recreates the shear force of the acetabular chondrolabral junction and reproduces symptoms.

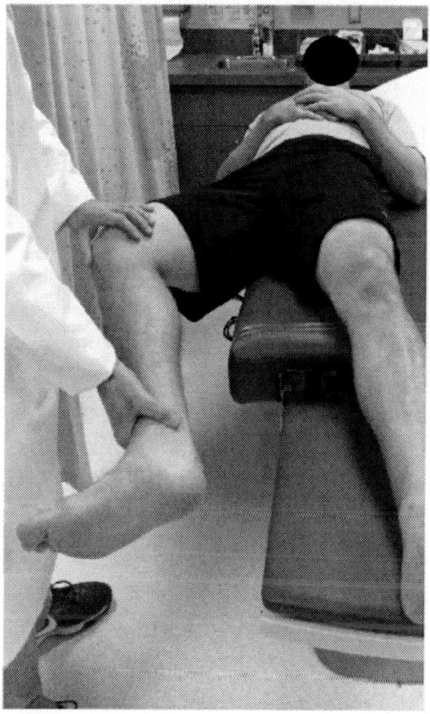

Figure 5. Posterior impingement is assessed with the patient supine and positioned with the involved leg off the table so that maximal external rotation and extension of the hip can be obtained.

Posterior impingement is less common but can be evaluated for by the examiner. It is tested with passive extension and external rotation of the involved hip (Figure 5). It is analogous to the anterior impingement test and comparison should be made between both extremities.

DIFFERENTIAL

The differential diagnosis for a young patient with hip pain is broad. A comprehensive history and physical is paramount to the differentiation of FAI from other pathologies causing anterior groin and hip pain. A brief overview of these pathologies is provided.

Snapping hip syndrome, or coxa saltans, is a relatively common condition that can present similarly to FAI. Coxa saltans can be divided into two types:

internal snapping hip, which generally occurs secondary to subluxation of the iliopsoas tendon over the anterior acetabular rim, and external snapping hip, which is caused by subluxation of the iliotibial band over the greater trochanter. (Schaberg, 1984). Coxa saltans is relatively common, particularly amongst patients with FAI. This is likely due to the fact that anterior acetabular prominence in patients with FAI may result in juxtaposition of the anterior rim to the tendon (Byrd, 2006). Consequently, when coxa saltans is encountered on exam, it is important to determine if the snapping is clinically symptomatic.

Athletic pubalgia, also known as sports hernia or core muscle injury, is another condition in athletes that presents with insidious groin pain. However, unlike FAI, symptoms arise from a weakened and dilated internal inguinal ring. Recent studies have recognized that patients with athletic pubalgia have an increased prevalence of coexistent hip disorders (Hammoud, 2012). Patients with FAI may compensate for loss of hip motion with increased movement through the pelvis, which may predispose them to the development of athletic pubalgia. Treatment should consist of surgical repair of the posterior inguinal wall, and concomitant hip pathology should be addressed concurrently or in staged fashion (Larson, 2011).

Osteitis pubis refers to inflammation of the pubic symphysis. Etiology of this condition is poorly understood, but is associated with vigorous athletic activity. Radiographic signs include erosive changes, sclerosis, and symphyseal irregularity. Treatment is symptomatic and includes activity modification, rest, and anti-inflammatory medications.

Other causes of hip pain include lumbar spine pathology, such as spondylolisthesis and herniated nucleus pulposus, adductor musculotendinous strain, iliac crest contusion (hip pointer), hip osteoarthritis, avascular necrosis of the femoral head, femoral neck stress fracture, and developmental dysplasia. The practitioner should be familiar with the respective diagnoses and management of these conditions.

Imaging

Plain Radiographs

General Considerations

Plain radiographs should be considered as an initial step in the diagnostic workup of athletes with persistent hip and groin pain (Clohisy, 2008).

Although radiographs may reveal findings related to conditions that cause symptoms similar to those of FAI such as osteitis pubis and femoral neck stress fractures, only those relevant to FAI are discussed.

It must be considered that radiographs are 2-dimensional representations of 3-dimensional anatomic structures. Thus, comprehensive characterization of pincer and cam deformities may be limited using plain radiographs alone. Advanced imaging, such as MRI, CT scan, and three-dimensional reconstructions should also be considered as a diagnostic adjunct. Additionally, poor intra-observer and inter-observer reliability of hip radiographs is reported in general, and images should be assessed in the context of athletes' complaints and exam findings (Clohisy 2009a). This is especially important, as FAI is a multidimensional process of which radiographic analysis is only one aspect of diagnostic and treatment decision-making algorithms.

Several radiographic views of the hip and pelvis are available to choose from, and the practitioner should be aware of the information provided by each. The anteroposterior radiograph is obtained with the patient supine and the lower extremities internally rotated 15° so as to maximize the femoral neck length visualized en face (Figure 6). Appropriate tilt is ensured by symmetry of the obturator foramina and proper inclination by a distance of approximately 2 cm from the caudal tip of the coccyx to the superior border of the pubic symphysis (Siebenrock, 2003) (Figure 7). The false-profile radiographic view is obtained by positioning the standing patient with the affected hip against the cassette (Figure 8). The ipsilateral foot is maintained parallel to the cassette, and the body is rotated 65° towards the beam. It is useful for assessment of anterior coverage of the femoral head. A cross-table lateral radiograph is taken with the patient supine, the limb of interest internally rotated 15°, the contralateral limb flexed greater than 80° at the hip and knee, and the beam oriented 45° obliquely to and centered at the femoral head of the limb of interest (Laage, 1953). The frog-leg lateral view is obtained with the patient supine; the knee of the extremity of interest is flexed 40° and the hip abducted 45° so that it assumes a "figure-4" position (Figure 9). The Dunn lateral view is taken with the patient supine. The hips are flexed 90°, abducted 15°, and held in neutral rotation. Both knees are also flexed 90° (Dunn, 1952) (Figure 10). This may alternatively be performed with the hips flexed 45°. Superimposition of the greater trochanter and femoral head-neck junction is common on the cross-table and frog-leg lateral radiographic views and may therefore prevent adequate assessment of cam deformities. The benefit of the Dunn lateral view is that obscuration of femoral head-neck junction by the greater trochanter is mitigated.

The radiographs of all patients suspected of having FAI should be inspected for the presence of osteoarthritis and congruency, as these have important implications for surgical intervention. In a normal, congruent hip, the roundness of the acetabulum matches that of the articulating portion of the femoral head. Either or both femoral and acetabular pathologic processes can result in loss of this congruence. Examples include Legg-Calve-Perthès disease, avascular necrosis, and acetabular developmental dysplasia. Such changes are classified according to the system proposed by Yasunaga et al. (2001) and are defined as excellent, good, fair, and poor.

The general radiographic characteristics of osteoarthritis are applicable to the hip and include: subchondral sclerosis, subchondral cyst formation, joint-space narrowing, and osteophyte formation (Tönnis, 1987).

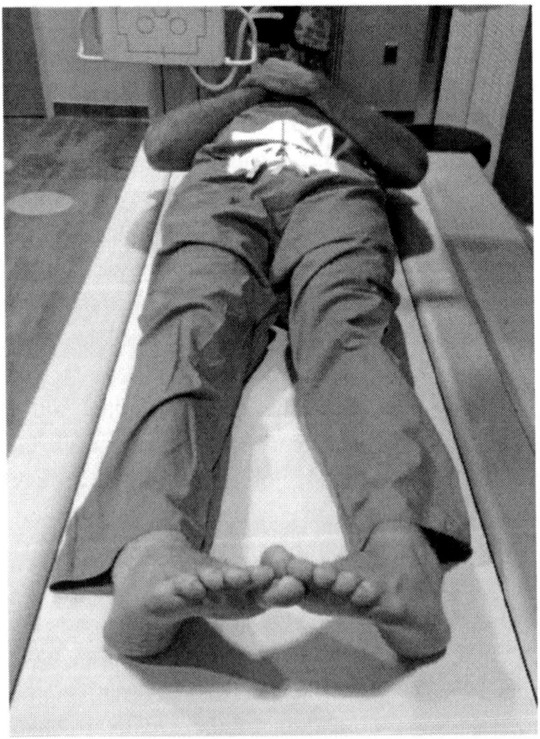

Figure 6. Anteroposterior radiographs are obtained with the patient supine and the lower extremities internally rotated 15° at the hip.

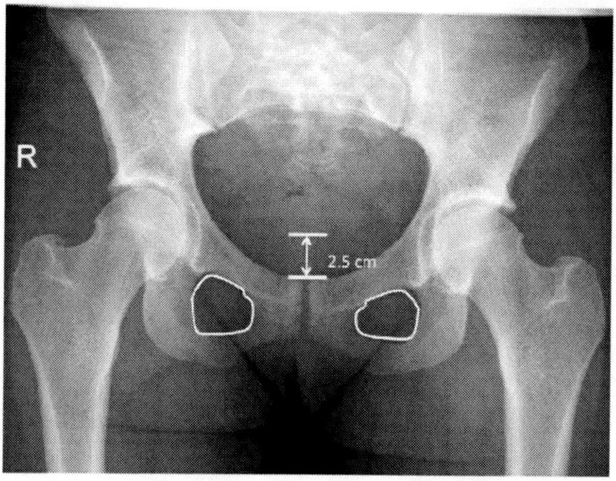

Figure 7. Anteroposterior radiograph is assessed for adequacy by a distance of approximately 2 cm from the coccyx to the superior pubic symphysis and symmetry of the obturator foramina.

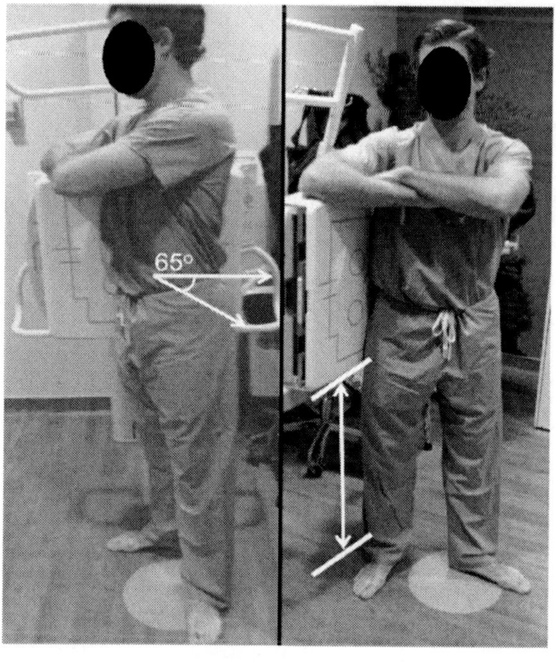

Figure 8. Technique of the false-profile view. The patient is positioned against the cassette and the foot of the adjacent extremity held parallel. The patient is then rotated 65° towards the beam.

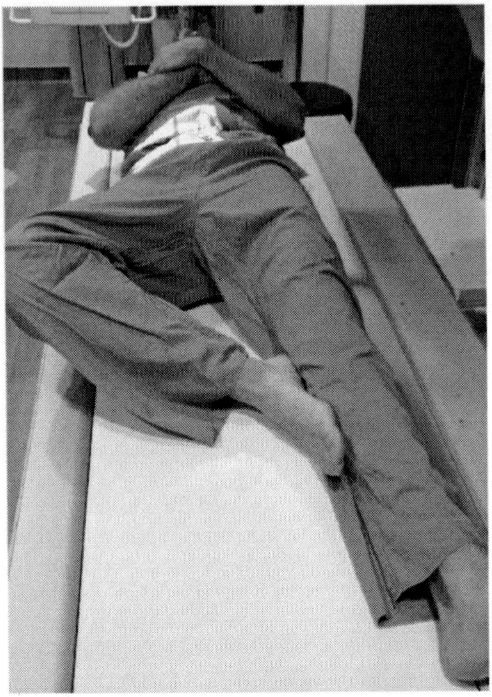

Figure 9. Patient positioning of the right leg for a frog-leg lateral view.

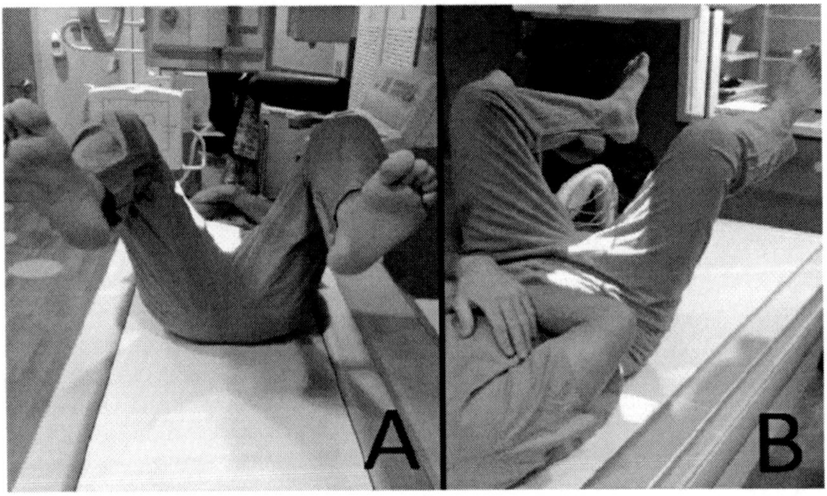

Figure 10. Patient positioning for the 90° Dunn lateral radiograph. (B) The beam is centered midway between the anterior superior iliac spine and pubic symphysis.

Pincer Deformity Evaluation

Pincer impingement is most pronounced and clinically relevant on the anterior acetabular rim. This can result from localized areas of bony protrusion or part of global acetabular overcoverage. There are several facets paramount to radiographic evaluation that must be considered in order to fully characterize the nature of the impingement. Acetabular depth, inclination, version, and formation of calcifications and ossified bodies all play a potential role and must be evaluated.

Global overcoverage may be associated with acetabular depth. This is assessed with reference to the ilioischial line on the anteroposterior view. If the acetabular wall extends to or beyond the ilioischial line medially, the hip is categorized as *coxa profunda. Protrusio acetabuli* is defined as extension of the medial aspect of the femoral head to or beyond the ilioischial line.

Measurement of the Tönnis angle is useful for determining acetabular inclination. It is the angle formed by a line drawn parallel to the horizontal pelvic axis and another line connecting the most inferior and lateral aspects of the sclerotic sourcil (Tönnis, 1987) (Figure 11). Normal values are considered 0° to 10°; greater values may confer risk of instability and lesser values risk of impingement. Acetabular coverage can also be assessed through other angular measurements on the various radiographic views (Wiberg, 1953). The center-edge angle of Wiberg is measured on an anteroposterior radiograph, and it is defined as the angle subtended by one line drawn parallel to the pelvic vertical axis through the center of the femoral head and another drawn from the center of the femoral head to the lateral-most point on the sourcil (Figure 11). Acetabular insufficiency is typically defined as a value less than 20° and over-coverage by a value greater than 40° (Wiberg, 1953; Jaberi, 2007). Assessment of anterior coverage, which is most clinically relevant to FAI, can best be made on the false-profile view by the Anterior Center-edge Angle, or Angle of Lequesne. It is defined as the angle formed from a vertical line extending from the center of the femoral head and another from the femoral head center to the most anterior point on the acetabular sourcil (Ganz 2003) (Figure 12). Other reliable indices have also been reported for estimating anterior coverage include the Anterior Acetabular Head Index, and the practitioner should be familiar with their preferred method (Chosa, 2003).

Acetabular version may also affect impingement symptoms. Retroversion is an anatomic variation in which the acetabular opening is oriented more posterolaterally than the normal anterolateral position.

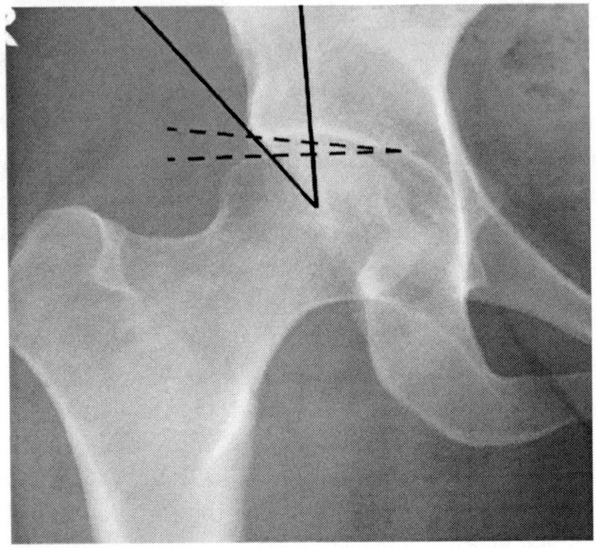

Figure 11. AP radiograph of the left hip demonstrating a normal Tönnis angle (dashed lines) and Center edge angle of Wiberg (solid lines).

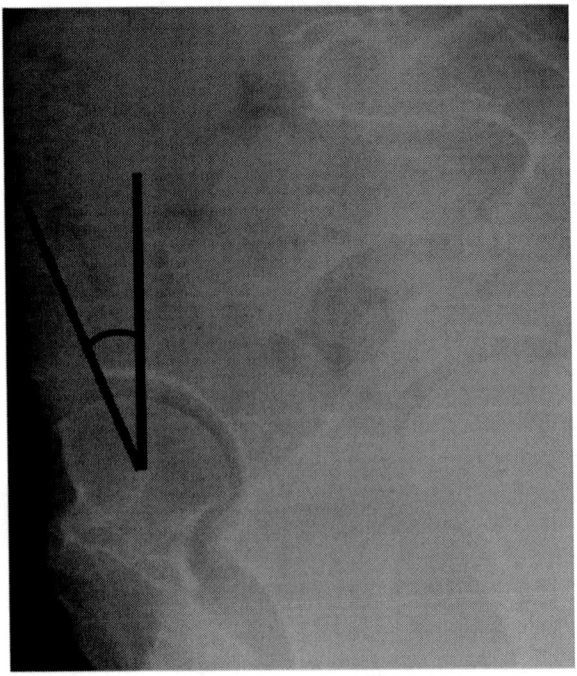

Figure 12. Center edge angle of Luquesne measured on the false profile view.

This may result in excessive anterior coverage and consequential impingement. It warrants discussion that acetabular retroversion implies anterior overcoverage and concomitant posterior wall deficiency. In the case of FAI, anterior overcoverage is most clinically salient and may be present without posterior deficiency due to localized bone formation. However, the term acetabular retroversion is still often used to refer to anterior overcoverage even in the absence posterior deficiency. Posterior wall deficiency may be evaluated on an adequate AP radiograph by assessing the relationship of the posterior wall line to the center of the femoral head. If the line is lateral to the center of the femoral head posterior wall overcoverage is likely, if it is medial to the femoral head, deficiency is present.

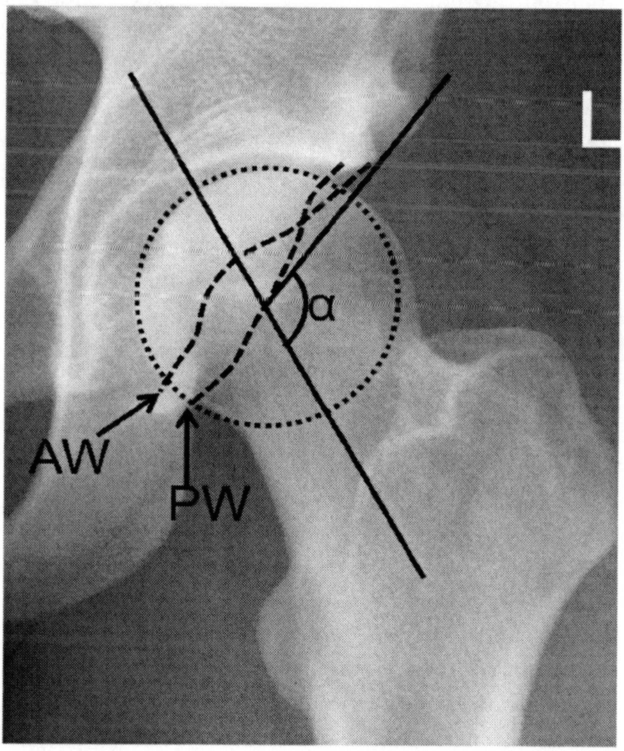

Figure 13. Anteroposterior radiograph of the left hip demonstrating the crossover sign (dashed lines) by crossing of the anterior wall (AW) over the posterior (wall). The alpha (α) angle is measured from by a line bisecting the femoral neck and center of the femoral head and another drawn from the center of the femoral head to the point where the radius of head-neck junction is greater than the articular portion. A large CAM lesions is seen here.

The crossover sign indicates overall and focal acetabular retroversion on anteroposterior radiographs (Figure 13). It is defined as the crossing of the anterior rim line over the posterior rim line before reaching the lateral sourcil (Jamali, 2007). However, this radiographic finding is affected by image orientation as well as anterior-inferior iliac spine morphology (Zaltz, 2013). Projection of the ischial spine into the pelvis is also associated with retroversion of the acetabulum (Kalberer, 2008).

The practitioner should note the presence of calcifications and osseous bodies about the hip joint. Calcifications that are visualized at the anterosuperior acetabulum have been implicated as pathophysiologic sequelae of repetitive impingement. Such trauma is theorized to incite a calcific response within the labrum and is therefore associated with FAI (Jackson, 2014). However, calcific tendonosis of the indirect head of the rectus femoris unrelated to FAI may also exhibit similar radiographic signs, and differentiation may be challenging (Sarkar, 1996). Osseous bodies in the same area may alternatively represent os acetabuli and/or rim fractures. Os acetabuli are defined as unfused accessory or secondary ossifying nuclei (Hergan, 2000). They are relatively common during adolescence and typically fuse by the end of the second decade of life. They can be found in the same area of the anterosuperior labrum, as well as in a variety of other locations within and surrounding the hip joint (Hergan, 2000).

Acetabular rim fractures are thought to represent a stress fracture resulting from repetitive abnormal contact with the femoral head (Larson, 2011; Epstein, 2009; Martinez, 2006). Differentiation of os acetabuli from rim fractures is often difficult given their similar appearance; however, the latter may be identified by a vertically oriented line of separation from the intact acetabulum, as opposed to a more horizontal demarcation in the case of os acetabuli (Martinez, 2006).

Cam Deformity Evaluation

A stepwise approach to assessing the femoral head and head-neck junction should be employed as it relates to FAI. Femoral head sphericity can be determined on any of the views but must be evaluated on at least two, as the head may appear spherical on an anteroposterior view but not on a lateral or vice-versa. Sphericity can be determined with gross visualization or more precisely with the use of concentric circles to which deviation of the joint surface is indicative of asphericity (Mose, 1980). This is independent of a cam deformity, which refers specifically to an osseous morphologic variation at the head-neck junction where a normal hip displays symmetric anterior and posterior concavity. It is typically most pronounced on the anterior head-neck junction between the 11:45 to 2:45 o'clock positions. For reference, the superior head-neck junction represents 12 o'clock and the anterior junction is referred to as the 3 o'clock position.

Three-dimensional imaging is the gold-standard for detecting cam lesions (Nepple, 2012b). The alpha angle, as initially described by Nötzli and colleagues (2002), was intended for use in assessing this deformity on tilted axial MR images. This angle is defined as that formed by a line connecting the point on the anterior femoral head-neck junction where the radius from the center of the femoral head exceeds that of the subchondral bone and another line connecting the femoral head center and the center of the narrowest point of the femoral neck (Nötzli, 2002) (Figure 13). A cam deformity is defined by many as any angle greater than 50.5° (Barton, 2011). Measurement of this angle on plain radiographs was subsequently described (Gosvig, 2007). However, reliability of this method has been questioned as radiograph projection, limb position, and femoral neck version all affect cam visualization (Meyer, 2006 Ross, 2014; Konan, 2010). To this end, several authors have investigated the reliability of radiographs for detection with various results; however, the Dunn lateral view is likely the most sensitive for this (Barton, 2011; Nepple, 2012b). Other authors suggest use of a series of radiographs including the AP, 45° Dunn lateral and frog-leg lateral views (Nepple, 2012b). Regardless of the views chosen, it is wise to assume that lesion severity is underestimated on plain radiographs compared to three-dimensional imaging (Konan, 2010, Nepple, 2012b). Additionally, fibrocystic changes localized to the anterosuperior aspect of the femoral neck as detected on anterosuperior radiographs may represent the consequence of repetitive contact with the anterior acetabulum and should also alert the practitioner to potential impingement (Leunig, 2005).

The clinical significance of radiographic signs of FAI is important to consider, as these deformities are also found in asymptomatic individuals (Hack, 2010; Kang, 2010). The prevalence of radiologic FAI in the asymptomatic general population has been reported as 17 - 24.7% for cam deformities in men, 2 – 5.4% for cam deformities in women, and 15.2% for pincer abnormalities, overall (Hack, 2010; Gosvig, 2008). However, there is a solid foundation of evidence that supports the association of clinical and radiologic impingement. For instance, the prevalence of radiologic FAI is greater in patients with hip pain that those without pain (Allen, 2009). Furthermore, larger cam lesions, as defined by the alpha angle, are associated with hip pain in the absence of arthritis and dysplasia (Allen, 2009).

Additionally, radiologic FAI is associated with the development of cartilage injury, labral tears, as well as the need for total hip arthroplasty in patients younger than 50 years (Bardakos, 2009; Wenger, 2004; Dolan, 2011; Van Thiel, 2013). Thus, the morphology of the acetabulum and proximal femoral head-neck junction very likely plays a significant role in the development of groin pain and progression of degenerative disease of the hip joint.

It is important to consider that anatomy of the hip joint is likely only one facet relevant to the development of symptomatic FAI in athletes. Athletes are often required to perform activities that involve hip movement at the passive limits, as well as in the supraphysiologic range for competition. Furthermore, osseous remodeling of the hip joint in response to increased loading has been suggested as an etiology for the development of FAI morphology (Galbraith 1987). Thus, repetitive movements commonly required for athletic performance that cause forceful abutment of the femur and acetabulum may affect the clinical relevance of radiologic FAI with regard to their severity and magnitude. To this end, several authors have investigated the prevalence of radiographic FAI in the athletic population. Gerhardt et al. (2012) reported radiographic hip abnormalities in 72% of male and 50% of female soccer players with groin pain. Larson and colleagues (2013) reported that larger cam deformities were an independent predictor of groin pain in National Football League prospects. A similar study revealed evidence of FAI in 94.3% of elite football players with a history of hip pain or injury (Nepple 2012a). Interestingly, another study evaluated asymptomatic collegiate football players for radiologic FAI and reported that 95% had at least one radiographic sign of FAI (Kapron 2011). Thus, although more severe radiologic FAI is associated with clinical impingement, these findings are also exceedingly common in the asymptomatic athlete.

MRI

MRI is advantageous in the assessment of FAI because of its multiplanar capabilities and detection of soft tissue and bony injuries. It also may aide in the identification of other pathologic processes with symptoms similar to those of FAI, such as bursitis, osteitis pubis, femoral neck stress fractures, femoral head osteonecrosis, and musculotendinous injuries. Most pertinent to FAI, the labrum, cartilage, and ligamentum teres may all be evaluated.

The optimal MR technique for the evaluation of FAI and its related pathology has not yet been established (Mamisch, 2008). Variables that should be considered when obtaining an MRI include image formatting, image resolution, and the use of gadolinium. Thus, communication between the practitioner and radiologist is paramount to ensure a protocol that facilitates detection of FAI and its related pathology is followed. Assessment of labral pathology and cam deformities made on standard coronal, sagittal, and axial views are less reliable than those made on radially reformatted images optimized for detection of labral pathology and evaluation of the head-neck junction (Ito, 2001; Kubo, 1999). Thus, these reformatted images should be obtained when possible, and consideration should also be given to preferentially ordering 3.0 Tesla (T) MRI tests to improve resolution and visualization of pertinent anatomic structures (Sundberg, 2006). The use of gadolinium contrast, which may be injected into the joint (direct MRA) or administered intravenously (indirect MRA), must also be considered. Direct MRA has consistently demonstrated superior detection of labral tears. The resultant distention from contrast injection defines the interval of the capsulolabral junction and permits filling of labral defects (Smith, 2011) (Figure 14). Local anesthetic can also be injected with gadolinium so that the practitioner can monitor any clinical response, as pain relief is a reliable indicator of intra-articular pathology (Byrd, 2004). However, intra-articular injection of contrast and anesthetic is an invasive procedure and is not without risk, such as neurovascular injury (Mamisch, 2008).

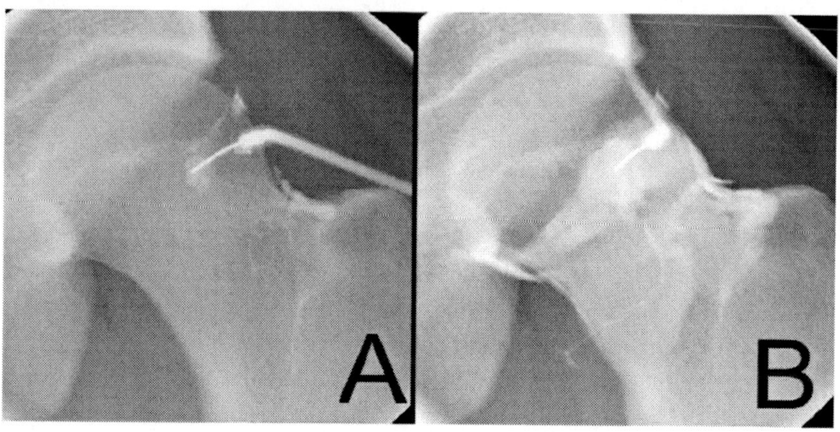

Figure 14. (A) Fluoroscopic image demonstrating the technique for injection gadolinium, anesthetic, and radiographic contrast. (B) Intra-articular placement is ensured by filling of the entire capsule.

The labrum typically has a diffusely dark, homogeneous triangular shape on MR images; however, normal variations have been reported and include sublabral sulci and acetabular clefts. Young, asymptomatic individuals may also reveal labral tears as indicated by linear high-signal extending to the joint surface (Schmitz, 2012). Despite these frequent variants, the reported sensitivity of labral pathology detection using direct and indirect MRA is 69 to 100% (Sutter, 2014; Zlatkin, 2010; Toomayan, 2006). The sensitivity of MRI for detection of cartilage pathology is low but evidence of chondral delamination as indicated by hypointensity of the chondral surface on T1 or intermediate-weighted, fat-saturated images has specificity approaching 100% (Pfirrmann, 2008; Anderson, 2009).

MRI is also useful for characterizing bony morphology of the femur and acetabulum. The gold-standard for evaluating cam-lesions is the alpha-angle as measured on radially reformatted MR images (Rakhra, 2009; Nötzli, 2002) (Figure 15). This is performed similarly to the method described for measurement on plain radiograph, and is made on a single image through the center of the femoral neck. First, a circle including the articular cartilage is drawn around the femoral head, next a line bisecting the circle and parallel to the longitudinal axis of the femoral neck at its narrowest point is made. The alpha-angle is formed by this line and another drawn from the circle's center to the point where the contour of the head-neck junction protrudes beyond the radius of the articulating surface of the femoral head. Measurements taken on axial oblique images underestimate the severity of the cam deformity and are less reliable than those from radial images (Rakhra, 2009). Regardless of the image that the alpha-angle is calculated, controversy still exists regarding the threshold that confers clinical significance (Sutter, 2012). Thus, alpha-angles must considered in the context of the entire clinical picture.

Acetabular version may be determined on the most cranial image that includes the femoral head. If the anterior acetabulum is medial to the posterior acetabular rim, the acetabulum is anteverted, and if the anterior rim is lateral to the posterior rim, the acetabulum is retroverted (Riley, 2014). Acetabular depth may be made on transverse oblique images through the center of the femoral neck. The distance between a line drawn tangential to the anterior and posterior acetabular rims and another drawn parallel through the center of the femoral head may reflect depth, and lower values are reflective of overcoverage (Pfirrmann, 2008). Additionally, the use biochemical MRI, which uses biomarkers to evaluate cartilage health prior to actual cartilage loss is also expanding and may be beneficial in the staging of FAI in the future (Siebenrock, 2014).

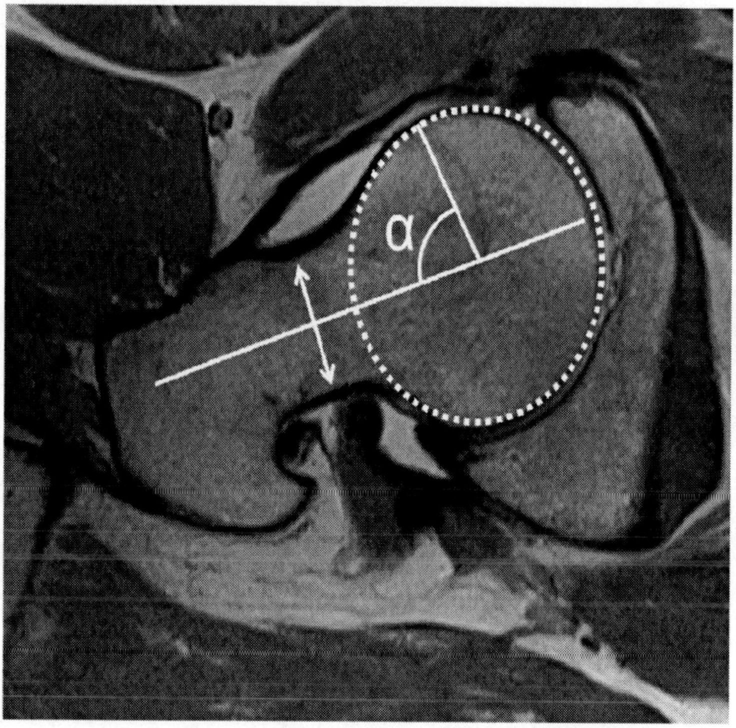

FIgure 15. Technique for assessing the alpha (α) angle on MR imaging.

Computed Tomography

CT may also be considered by the practitioner for characterization of FAI. Although CT does not provide information regarding labrum and cartilage injury, it is helpful in the evaluation of bony morphology (Milone, 2013). Typically, CT is used when assessment of the bony anatomy on plain radiographs is inconclusive or reveals borderline deformities, as well as instances of severe deformity for the purposes of operative planning. Three-dimensional (3-D) reformatted images may also be acquired using CT, which provide surface renderings of the hip joint for accurate assessment of cam and pincer deformities using topographic representations (Figure 16). The hip joint may be placed in a position of maximal discomfort (flexion, adduction, and internal rotation) during image acquisition to more precisely identify areas of problematic impingement (Grabinski, 2014). Additionally, CT also provides for more accurate assessment of herniation pits, which helps the practitioner to localize the areas of greatest abutment (Panzer, 2008).

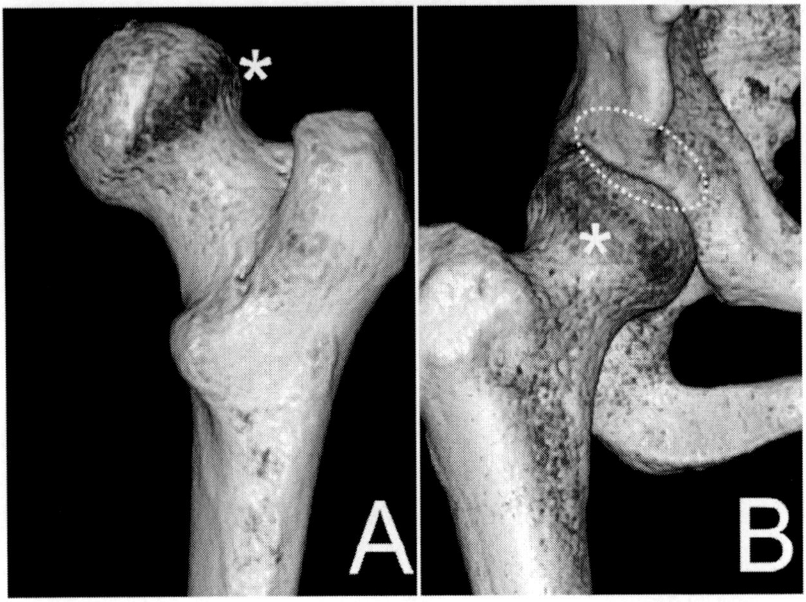

Figure 16. Three-dimensional reformatted CT rendering of a borderline cam and pincer lesions. (A) small area of cam-deformity (*) is evident on the anterosuperior head-neck junction from the posterior view. (B) small pincer-type deformity (*) is present on the anterolateral acetabulum.

Prevention

There are no recommendations regarding the prevention of FAI. However, the basic principles of disease prevention can be reasonably applied to our current understanding of FAI in order to establish a framework to develop such guidelines. This is a worthwhile endeavor, particularly in the athletic population, given that FAI is associated with the acceleration of osteoarthritis progression, disability, pain, and decreased range of motion. Success in this regard is dependent upon knowledge of causation, identification of risk, availability of early detection and effective prophylaxis or treatment, as well as a means to apply such measures. Prevention is best evaluated in the context of the following discrete levels: primordial, primary, secondary, and tertiary.

Primordial prevention refers to inhibition of the emergence of environmental and behavioral risk factors. Risk factors for the development of FAI, particularly cam deformities, are theorized to include slipped capital femoral epiphysis (SCFE), vigorous adolescent athletic participation, and certain repetitive physical maneuvers (Klit, 2014; Castañeda, 2013, Wensaas, 2012). Thus, with regards to SCFE, primordial preventative measures should be directed towards modifiable risk factors for its development. This includes controlling childhood obesity and clearly defining indications for prophylactic pinning (Nasreddine, 2013).

Pediatric and adolescent participation in sports must also be evaluated. A causal relationship between altered proximal femoral morphology as it relates to osteoarthritis and adolescent athletic participation was suggested as early as 1971 by Murray and Duncan. There is a growing body of evidence that likewise suggests cam deformities develop during physeal closure and are related to an increased activity level during this period (Carsen, 2014; Siebenrock, 2013a). Along these lines, elite-level adolescent basketball players exhibit a higher prevalence of cam-type deformities compared to non-athletes. This has been demonstrated by increased epiphyseal extension, which is characterized by an abnormal capital physeal shape prior to its closure, and increased alpha angles in the skeletally mature (Siebenrock, 2013a). Similarly, adolescent male basketball players exhibit a 10-fold risk of having an alpha angle greater than 55^{0} compared to non-athletes (Siebenrock, 2013a). They also exhibit less internal rotation (Siebenrock, 2011). Philippon and colleagues (2013b) demonstrated that youth hockey players were 4.5 times more likely to have an alpha angle greater than 55^{0} compared to a matched cohort of skiers. There was also significant correlation between alpha angle severity and increasing age, which the control group did not exhibit. The authors concluded that participation in ice hockey contributed to the development of cam deformities. The clinical significance of this is illustrated by the fact that adolescent male ice hockey players with larger cam deformities are more likely to have hip pain and decreased range of motion (Siebenrock, 2013b). These findings in total suggest that vigorous athletic activity during growth and physeal closure may alter the physis itself and contribute to altered hip morphology. Consequently, the pathomechanism of cam-type deformities may be developmental and not the result of reactive bone formation.

It is unclear if these anatomic changes may result from the cumulative effect of overall repetitive abnormal stresses or from specific physical maneuvers. In support of the latter, unique positions commonly assumed in certain sports such as ice hockey that increase the likelihood of impingement have been identified. These include abduction and external rotation during the push-off phase of a hockey stride and flexion and internal rotation at termination of the recovery phase (Stull, 2011). Youth players demonstrate these biomechanics, which may potentially increase the risk of developing intra-articular pathology and promoting the formation of cam and pincer deformities (Stull, 2011). Conversely, although the repetitive movement required of female ballet dancers often cause painful femoroacetabular abutment, the prevalence of FAI morphology is lower than in other athletes and more likely to be a pincer-type deformity (Duthon, 2013; Kolo, 2013). Primordial prevention in light of these findings could include avoidance of certain high-risk athletic activities in general or limited abstinence during vulnerable phases of development in particular. However, further research is needed to make specific recommendations, which would also require consideration of the benefits of athletic participation.

Primary prevention refers to actions directed towards eliminating the possibility of disease occurrence. Facets of this stage include positive health promotion to facilitate patient control over potential detriments of health and implementation of targeted protective measures. In the case of FAI, this may include athlete, parent, and coach education to increase awareness that adolescent strenuous athletic participation may predispose the athlete to developing hip pathology. However, until it is determined whether athletic participation overall may induce the formation of FAI morphology or if it is only certain physical maneuvers required in some sports that play the primary developmental role, such recommendations cannot be made. For instance, if is determined that FAI results from overuse due to strenuous athletic participation, devising guidelines analogous to those established by the USA Baseball Medical and Safety Advisory Committee for pitching athletes would be useful. If it was found that it only certain physical maneuvers confer risk for the development of FAI, then biomechanic adjustments would be advisable. For example, in the case of youth hockey, in which athletes repetitively posture their hips in "at-risk" positions during play, adjustments in training drills, such as skating exercises with resistance bands, would be advisable (Stull, 2011). Similarly, a trend towards greater FAI-type morphology has been found in players of football positions that require greater repetitive forceful flexion, such as tight-end and lineman (Nepple, 2012). Additionally, soccer players display greater alpha angles on their kicking leg compared to their non-kicking leg, and elite-level players have greater alpha angles than their amateur counterparts (Lahner, 2014b). Thus, consideration may be given to promoting and training with altered biomechanics. However, additional research is clearly required before evidence-based recommendations can be made in this regard.

Development and institution of protective equipment represents an alternative avenue to prevention at the primary stage. A basis for this intervention can be envisioned by the theory that certain repetitive physical maneuvers result in impingement morphology. Thus, equipment that inhibits or modifies such motion and posture may be beneficial. For instance, ice hockey goaltenders are required to assume a butterfly position, which places the hips at the maximum limits of internal rotation with their legs resting parallel on the ice (Wijdicks, 2014). Goaltender leg pad wear has been shown to affect hip kinematics in this position, and may therefore influence the development of FAI morphology (Wijdicks, 2014).

Secondary prevention attempts to inhibit progression of disease and implement treatment before irreversible pathologic changes take place. Goals of secondary prevention in the case of FAI would be to reduce incidence of labral and chondral damage from impingement as well as the progression of osteoarthritis. A screening program for athletes at risk for developing future hip pathology would serve this goal. Currently, the South African Society of Hip Arthroscopy is implementing such a program with the use of clinically proven manual tests to assess hip function and signs of impingement (Cakic, 2014). Unfortunately, it is impossible to establish recommendations regarding further diagnostic workup or intervention based on information garnered by such programs at this point. It should also be noted that although evidence supports using arthroscopic techniques to improve impingement type symptoms, their role in preventing osteoarthritis has not been fully elucidated (Clohisy, 2010). This is particularly relevant in the athletic population, as elite male and female athletes are at higher risk for developing hip osteoarthritis than the general population (Tveit, 2012; Vingård, 1993 & 1998). Such programs are in their nascent stage, and a protocol to monitor these at-risk athletes is far from established. Questions that will need to be answered include: (1) Should asymptomatic patients with impingement based on examination be monitored radiographically?; (2) Should asymptomatic patients with clinical and radiologic FAI be referred for intervention?; and if so, (3) which interventions are indicated?

Another facet to consider with regards to prevention is whether decreased hip range of motion, specifically internal rotation, may potentially predispose the athlete to compensatory hip disorders (Nepple, 2012). Additionally, it is entirely possible that athletes with FAI are at increased risk for developing other injuries all together. Along this line, soccer players with higher alpha angles exhibit altered gait mechanics that increase loading across the lower extremity and may theoretically predispose soccer players to injury elsewhere in the extremity (Lahner, 2014a).

Tertiary prevention includes interventions to limit disability and promote rehabilitation once the disease has advanced beyond early stages. In the case of FAI, focus is elimination of impingement to mitigate cartilage labral damage and stave off progression of osteoarthritis. This will be discussed in further detail in the treatment section.

TREATMENT

Nonoperative Management

There is no nonoperative treatment that can alter the bony morphology relevant to FAI. However, because cam and pincer type deformities are only one component of symptomatic impingement, it may be possible to implement conservative techniques that effectively aide in symptom and pain management, as well as control of motion and activities that provoke impingement and damage intraarticular structures. Although conservative management is typically advocated as the initial approach in patients with FAI, this is largely based on opinion and convention. There is a dearth of high-quality evidence in this regard with few exception (Wall, 2013). Nonetheless, a course of nonoperative management is typically recommended for patients with FAI, and the practitioner should be familiar with the components of a successful algorithm.

In general, the basic concepts of conservative treatment of any musculoskeletal disorder have been extrapolated to the management of FAI. This includes relative rest and use of non-steroid anti-inflammatories (NSAIDs) during periods of acute exacerbation and worsening pain, modification of and abstinence from provocating activities, and physical therapy aimed at correcting hip biomechanics salient to FAI. The goals of the lattermost intervention include balancing of the musculature about the hip, followed by strengthening of the muscles to promote biomechanically-sound movement specific to individuals' normal activities. It is important for the practitioner, patient, and therapist to understand that improved range of motion is not a goal of treatment and should not be expected.

To this end, one study by Emara et al. (2011) reported improved function and symptoms so long as individuals were able to modify their activities of daily living to accommodate their hip morphology. The authors utilized a four-stage approach. This included: 1) avoidance of excessive activity and judicious use of NSAIDs; 2) physical therapy and stretching; 3) identification of a safe range of motion in which impingement does not occur; 4) modification of activities of daily living to reflect the safe range of motion. In this cohort, only 4 of 37 patients went on to require surgery during the 25 to 28 month follow-up period. Hunt et al. (2012) reported similar outcomes using a protocol that

Table 1. Tönnis Grade of Osteoarthritis

Tönnis Grade	Radiographic Characteristics
0	Normal; No arthritis evident
1	Acetabular and femoral head sclerosis, minimal joint space narrowing, and slight lipping at the joint margins
2	Small acetabular and femoral head cysts with moderate joint space narrowing and loss of sphericity
3	Large cyst formation, severe joint space narrowing or obliteration, as well as evidence of osteonecrosis.

Table 2. Key Components of Physical Therapy Protocol (adapted from Hunt D, Prather H, Harris Hayes M, Clohisy JC. Clinical outcomes analysis of conservative and surgical treatment of patients with clinical indications of prearthritic, intra-articular hip disorders. PM R 2012;4:479-87.)

PRECAUTIONS	GOALS
No straight leg raises	Improve hip motion precision
Exercises that require only pain-free motion	Prevent hip hyperextension with motion
Avoidance of acetabular and femoral rotation under axial loading	Prevent acetabular and femoral rotation under axial loading
Avoidance of hyperextension during exercise or other activities	Optimize hamstring length without pain during modalities
Avoidance of anterior femoral translation	Balance of hamstring and quadriceps
	Improve iliopsoas, gluteus maximus, gluteus medius, intrinsic hip lateral rotators (if not short), and abdominals performance
	Decrease anterior femoral glide with muscular retraining
	Education for modification of daily activities
	Home exercise program

incorporated activity modification, patient education, and directed physical therapy. The goals of therapy were specific and included exercises aimed at optimizing muscular function about the hip joint to limit anterior femoral glide (Table 2). Approximately, half of the cohort was sufficiently satisfied with conservative care that they did not require operative intervention at 1 year. The authors concluded that a trial of conservative therapy is worthwhile in individuals with pre-arthritic hip conditions, which include FAI (Hunt, 2012). Despite these results, however, the effect of conservative therapy on athletes' ability to return to sport remains to be seen, and careful monitoring of clinical status and playing performance is advisable in the case of the young active individual.

Surgical Intervention

There are no formal indications for surgical intervention in the patient with FAI. Typically, however, surgery is recommend for individuals with recalcitrant or worsening pain with evidence of radiologic FAI. The goals of surgery for the treatment of FAI are to address intraarticular pathology with a focus on the cartilage and labrum and prevention of future impingement with resection and/or correction of offending bony anatomy. Essentially, two surgical options exist in general, open and arthroscopic based procedures. Decisions regarding the surgical approach are largely based on surgeon and patient preference, as well as the nature of the pathology as characterized on preoperative imaging.

As previously mentioned, comprehensive assessment of the bony morphology is imperative to determine the areas of the femur and acetabulum that are causing impingement so that resection can be performed precisely. The cam-deformity is typically present on the anterosuperior aspect of the head-neck junction from the 12:00 to 2:00 o'clock positions; however, these deformities may extend posteriorly and may not be amenable to arthroscopic based procedures (Nepple, 2013; Matsuda, 2013). Likewise, preoperative characterization of the pincer lesion is required. Consideration must be given to the various facets of acetabular morphology relevant to impingement, which are version, inclination, depth, and localized abnormal bone formation. In the case of a truly retroverted acetabulum with anterior overcoverage and posterior deficiency, a periacetabular osteotomy may be most indicated (Siebenrock, 2003; Sierra, 2013). However, reports of this technique for the management of FAI are limited. Conversely, the more typical pattern of localized acetabular anterosuperior overcoverage with normal posterior coverage is amenable to trimming of the affected acetabular rim either with open or arthroscopic based procedures.

The presence of arthritis must also be evaluated and is an important consideration in these preservation techniques, as those with more advanced arthritis have worse outcomes. To this end, Philippon et al. (2013a) determined that a joint space of 2 mm or less was predictive of arthroscopic failure and progression to total hip arthroplasty 80% of the time in patients older than 50 years. The surgeon should also use caution when considering arthroscopy for patients with DDH, as iatrogenic destabilization and progression of osteoarthritis following arthroscopic procedures have been reported and are potentially catastrophic (Mei-Dan, 2012; Parvizi, 2009).

Open Surgical Treatment

Open treatment of FAI was initially described by Ganz et al. (2001) through a surgical dislocation. This procedure is conducted in the lateral decubitus position. A trochanteric osteotomy is performed through a Kocher-Langenbach approach, followed by a Z-shaped capsulotomy that is always kept anterior to the lesser trochanter. This allows for anterior dislocation of the hip and 360° visualization of the acetabulum and femoral head. Success of this technique is dependent on preservation of the blood supply of the femoral head by avoiding disruption to the medial femoral circumflex artery, which is protected by the obturator externus during dislocation (Ganz, 2001; Gautier, 2000). In their initial report, Ganz and colleagues (2001) reported no cases of osteonecrosis, and these results have been corroborated (Sink, 2011). However, the authors did report complications of partial sciatic neuropraxia, failure of trochanteric fixation, heterotopic ossification (37%), and a saddleback deformity at the incision (Ganz, 2001).

Outcomes of open treatments for FAI have generally been successful. In the short-term, functional improvement and pain relief have been reported; however, the benefit of this surgical strategy is less in those with more advanced cartilage disease (Peters, 2006 & 2010). Successful outcomes have also been reported with femoral osteochondroplasty of the cam deformity using an open approach (Bealué, 2007). Likewise, the open approach provides for successful acetabular rim resection and management of the labrum, with improved outcomes associated with refixation of the labrum as opposed to debridement only (Espinosa, 2006). Midterm results have also been positive overall; however, older, thinner female patients have been reported by some to be more likely to require conversion to THA or additional revision surgery

(Naal, 2012). Beck et al. (2004) reported similar results at an average follow-up of 4.7 years and additionally reported that the presence of degenerative changes was associated with worse outcomes. Steppacher and colleagues (2014) performed an investigation to elucidate factors associated with poorer outcomes following surgical hip dislocation and identified that excessive acetabular trimming, increased age, and weight were all associated with inferior clinical outcomes and progression to OA. With regards to athletes in particular, surgical hip dislocations have been shown to achieve reduced pain and improvement in activity level (Novais, 2014). Similar results have also been reported in professional athletes (Naal, 2011). While long-term results are lacking, open treatment for FAI offers promising results including the athletic population and warrant consideration by the practitioner and patient.

Of course no procedure is without potential complications. In a multicenter study examining the complications associated with surgical dislocations of the hip, the overall incidence was 9% and 4.8% if cases of heterotopic ossification were excluded (Sink, 2011). Persistent pain at the trochanteric osteotomy site is likely the most frequently encountered complication and is most prevalent amongst females; however, it does not appear to affect overall clinical outcomes, as opposed to persistent groin pain which does proted inferior results (Beck, 2011). The origin of the trochanteric pain is unclear; however bursitis associated with hardware fixation has been implicated in at least some of the cases, and it may be amenable to screw removal once union is obtained (Bealué, 2007). The patient should be counseled regarding these risks, especially given the relatively high incidence of pain at the greater trochanter, which could be particularly problematic in the athletic population.

Arthroscopy

Hip arthroscopy preceded the identification of FAI as a distinct entity. However, as recognition and understanding of FAI has expanded, so have the number of arthroscopic procedures of the hip (Colvin, 2012). In fact, an eighteen-fold increase in the number of arthroscopic hip procedures performed has been estimated over a 10-year period from 1999 to 2009 (Colvin, 2012). Despite the increasing popularity of hip arthroscopy, the indications and limitations of this procedure continue to be defined.

Hip arthroscopy is typically performed in the supine position, with the assistance of traction provided by specific operating tables and attachments. The first portal that is established is generally the primary viewing portal, the anterolateral portal, and is made under fluoroscopic guidance. Additional portals are made as indicated for instrumentation and include the posterolateral, anterior, distal anterolateral, and mid-anterior portals. This method allows for direct inspection of the both the central compartment of the joint and the peripheral compartment, which contains the head-neck junction where cam-deformities are present.

Arthroscopy allows for management of cartilage, labrum, and bony pathology. Labral pathology should be addressed prior to cartilage lesions, as the chondrolabral junction is usually most affected and labral stabilization may also secure adjacent delaminated cartilage. Options for management of labral tears includes debridement, repair, and reconstruction. Debridement is typically performed with an arthroscopic shaver to remove diseased, frayed, and loose tissue. Repair is performed with the use of suture anchors to pull back and stabilize the labrum to the underlying acetabulum **(Figure 17)**. Reconstruction is performed with the use of a tissue graft, typically iliotibial band, in instances in which repair is not possible and the individual's activity level should require it.

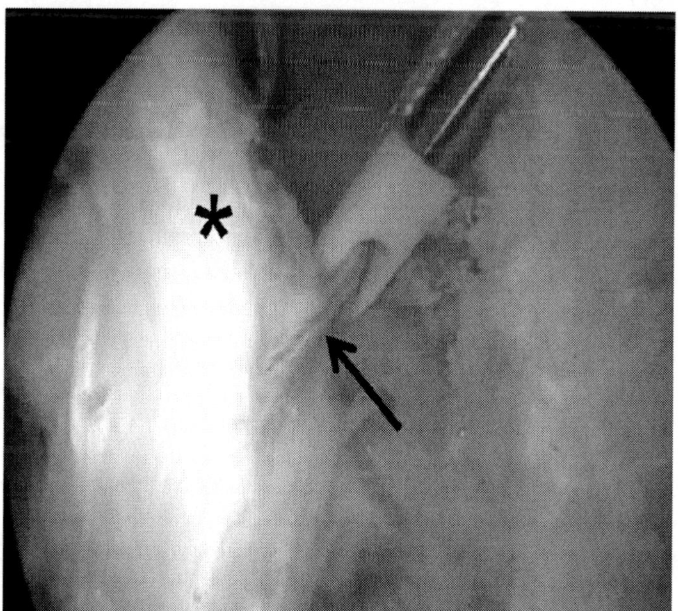

Figure 17. Arthroscopic view of labral repair using a suture anchor. A suture (arrow) has been passed through the labrum (*) and a suture anchor to be secured to the acetabular rim.

There is no consensus on the indications for any of these techniques, and a recent review of the literature was unable to make any definitive conclusions due to the small number of studies available and their heterogeneity (Haddad, 2014). The authors did offer that repair of a tear in an otherwise good quality labrum is logical; however, debridement may be a better option in individuals with degenerative pathology where preservation of the labrum is unlikely to restore its physiologic function (Haddad, 2014). This is consistent with the results of other comparative studies (Schilders, 2011). In the case of young, active individuals, whose labrums would be expected to be of healthier quality, repair is associated with improved clinical results (Larson, 2012). For those athletes, in which repair is not possible, reconstruction of the labrum with iliotibial band graft may also be considered as opposed to debridement or resection (Boykin, 2013; Geyer, 2013).

Several options exist for the management of cartilage injuries that are typically in the form of delamination from the underlying subchondral bone. These include debridement, debridement and microfracture, and reattachment with fibrin sealant (Stafford, 2011). Microfracture is performed with the goal of promoting fibrocartilage filling of chondral defects through bone marrow stimulation and release of pluripotent mesenchymal cells from the underlying subchondral bone. It may be performed with an awl or a flexible drill (Figure 18). This technique has been found to provide excellent coverage of cartilage defects and is associated with improved clinical outcomes (Karthikeyan, 2012; Philippon, 2008). It has also demonstrated good outcomes in elite level athletes as well, with 77% returning to play following microfracture (McDonald, 2013 & 2014). Osteochondroplasty of the cam-deformities can also be performed arthroscopically. This is performed with the extremity free of traction and use of an arthroscopic bur. Dynamic assessment is also possible to ensure that sufficient bone has been removed.

The ability for athletes to return to sport following arthroscopic based procedures is very good (Nho, 2011; Alradwan, 2012; Singh, 2010). One systematic review found a return rate of 92% with 88% achieving their previous level of competition (Alradwan, 2012). This provides valuable information for the practitioner when counseling the young athletic population on surgical options.

Although arthroscopy is less invasive than open-type procedures, it is not without potential complications. The overall complication rate is typically estimated to be approximately 5% (Sampson, 2001; Clarke, 2003).

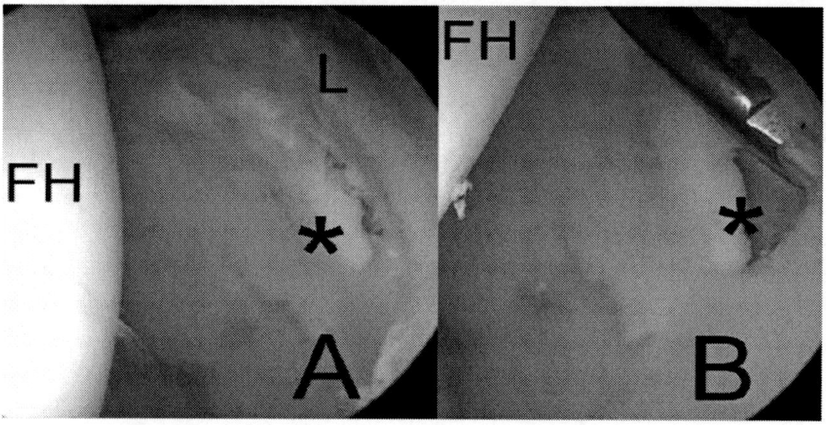

Figure 18. (A) Arthroscopic view of a large cartilage lesion (*) on the superior dome of the acetabulum. FH = Femoral head, L – Labrum. (B) Microfracture using a flexible drill through the defect (*).

However, it is very likely that iatrogenic cartilage and labral injury is underreported. The most common complication that has been reported is neuropraxia. It is typically the sequelae of prolonged traction during the procedure; the pudendal nerve is most commonly involved nerve (Park, 2014; Harris, 2013). Major complications have also been reported and include intra-abdominal compartment syndrome, femoral neck fracture, and avascular necrosis (Bardakos, 2012; Fowler, 2010; Tannast, 2008).

Multiple nonsurgical and surgical options exist for the management of FAI, but an algorithm to guide optimal management has yet to be defined. Comparison of arthroscopic procedures to open procedures is lacking; however, one report found a quicker recovery and return to sport with arthroscopic-based procedures (Botser, 2014). Others have demonstrated greater satisfaction with regards to sports that persists at 2 years following surgery using arthroscopic techniques compared to open ones (Domb, 2013). Comparison of long-term results of the two procedures is still lacking, however, and in the absence of firm indications to guide surgical management, operative decisions should be based upon surgeon and patient preferences.

Rehabilitation

Successful outcomes of FAI surgery require a comprehensive and effective rehabilitative protocol. This cannot be achieved through a single approach, but requires a program tailored on an individual basis. Several basic concepts should establish the framework for these programs, and the general principles of rehabilitation following hip arthroscopy include: 1) individualization of rehabilitation programs based on surgical findings and patient goals; 2) early mobility in the form of circumduction to prevent scar tissue formation; 3) sport-specific protocols for the athletic population (Wahoff, 2011). Throughout the process, consideration of pain control, reduction in muscle inhibition, restoration of proprioception, improved strength should all be given. Additionally, in the athlete, focus on agility, power, and speed should also be provided (Wahoff, 2011). A recent study found that most athletes were satisfied with their ability to return to sport despite having some limitations but were dissatisfied with their rehabilitation process, citing that physical therapy input was insufficient (Lovett Carter, 2013). Thus, there is also room for improvement in establishing the optimal rehabilitation process for patients that have undergone operative management of FAI. Future research is needed in this regard.

CONCLUSION

FAI represents a challenging problem for the athlete, orthopaedic surgeon, physical therapist, family, and coach. Paramount to effective management of FAI, is an in-depth understanding of the relationship between FAI morphology, patient activity and movement, and intraarticular injury. It is only through careful radiologic evaluation and clinical examination that effective treatment strategies can be implemented on an individual basis. Management should first proceed with nonoperative modalities, as well as patient education regarding the probable association between FAI and the development of OA later in life. Surgical intervention is warranted in the patient with recalcitrant pain despite implementation of nonoperative modalities. Patients should be counseled on both the potential complications of surgery as well as the likelihood of returning to sport. Undoubtedly, an effective rehabilitative protocol is required and should be individualized and progressed based on frequent clinical evaluation. As our understanding of the pathogenesis of FAI expands, the next step in the management of FAI should be implementation of prevention strategies, as well as improvement of diagnostic modalities, staging, surgical indications, and the rehabilitative process.

REFERENCES

Allen D, Beaule PE, Ramadan O, Doucette S. Prevalence of associated deformities and hip pain in patients with cam-type femoroacetabular impingement. *J Bone Joint Surg Br* 2009;91:589-94

Alradwan H, Philippon MJ, Farrokhyar F, et al. Return to preinjury activity levels after surgical management of femoroacetabular impingement in athletes. *Arthroscopy* 2012;28:1567-76.

Anderson LA, Peters CL, Park BB, Stoddard GJ, Erickson JA, Crim JR. Acetabular cartilage delamination in femoroacetabular impingement. Risk factors and magnetic resonance imaging diagnosis. *J Bone Joint Surg Am* 2009;91:305-13.

Bardakos NV, Papavasiliou AV. Death after fluid extravasation in hip arthroscopy. *Arthroscopy* 2012;28:1584; author reply.

Bardakos NV, Villar RN. Predictors of progression of osteoarthritis in femoroacetabular impingement: a radiological study with a minimum of ten years follow-up. *J Bone Joint Surg Br* 2009;91:162-9.

Barton C, Salineros MJ, Rakhra KS, BeaulÈ PE. Validity of the alpha angle measurement on plain radiographs in the evaluation of cam-type femoroacetabular impingement. *Clin Orthop Relat Res* 2011;469:464-9.

Beaulé PE, Le Duff MJ, Zaragoza E. Quality of life following femoral head-neck osteochondroplasty for femoroacetabular impingement. *J Bone Joint Surg Am* 2007;89:773-9.

Beck M, B¸chler L. Prevalence and impact of pain at the greater trochanter after open surgery for the treatment of femoro-acetabular impingement. *J Bone Joint Surg Am* 2011;93 Suppl 2:66-9.

Beck M, Kalhor M, Leunig M, Ganz R. Hip morphology influences the pattern of damage to the acetabular cartilage: femoroacetabular impingement as a cause of early osteoarthritis of the hip. *J Bone Joint Surg Br* 2005;87:1012-8.

Beck M, Leunig M, Parvizi J, Boutier V, Wyss D, Ganz R. Anterior femoroacetabular impingement: part II. Midterm results of surgical treatment. *Clin Orthop Relat Res* 2004:67-73.

Botser IB, Jackson TJ, Smith TW, Leonard JP, Stake CE, Domb BG. Open surgical dislocation versus arthroscopic treatment of femoroacetabular impingement. *Am J Orthop (Belle Mead NJ)* 2014;43:209-14.

Boykin RE, Patterson D, Briggs KK, Dee A, Philippon MJ. Results of arthroscopic labral reconstruction of the hip in elite athletes. *Am J Sports Med* 2013;41:2296-301.

Byrd JW. Evaluation and management of the snapping iliopsoas tendon. *Instr Course Lect* 2006;55:347-55.

Byrd JW. Femoroacetabular impingement in athletes: current concepts. *Am J Sports Med* 2014;42:737-51.

Byrd JW, Jones KS. Diagnostic accuracy of clinical assessment, magnetic resonance imaging, magnetic resonance arthrography, and intra-articular injection in hip arthroscopy patients. *Am J Sports Med* 2004;32:1668-74.

Byrd JW, Jones KS. Arthroscopic femoroplasty in the management of cam-type femoroacetabular impingement. *Clin Orthop Relat Res* 2009a;467:739-46.

Byrd JW, Jones KS. Arthroscopic management of femoroacetabular impingement. *Instr Course Lect* 2009b;58:231-9.

Cakic J, Patricios J. Femoroacetabular impingement: prevention or intervention? The sports physician's quandary. *Br J Sports Med* 2014;48:1073-4.

Carsen S, Moroz PJ, Rakhra K, et al. The Otto Aufranc Award. On the etiology of the cam deformity: a cross-sectional pediatric MRI study. *Clin Orthop Relat Res* 2014;472:430-6.

Castañeda P, Ponce C, Villareal G, Vidal C. The natural history of osteoarthritis after a slipped capital femoral epiphysis/the pistol grip deformity. *J Pediatr Orthop* 2013;33 Suppl 1:S76-82.

Chosa E, Tajima N. Anterior acetabular head index of the hip on false-profile views. New index of anterior acetabular cover. *J Bone Joint Surg Br* 2003;85:826-9.

Clarke MT, Arora A, Villar RN. Hip arthroscopy: complications in 1054 cases. *Clin Orthop Relat Res* 2003:84-8.

Clohisy JC, Carlisle JC, BeaulÈ PE, et al. A systematic approach to the plain radiographic evaluation of the young adult hip. *J Bone Joint Surg Am* 2008;90 Suppl 4:47-66.

Clohisy JC, Carlisle JC, Trousdale R, et al. Radiographic evaluation of the hip has limited reliability. *Clin Orthop Relat Res* 2009a;467:666-75.

Clohisy JC, Knaus ER, Hunt DM, Lesher JM, Harris-Hayes M, Prather H. Clinical presentation of patients with symptomatic anterior hip impingement. *Clin Orthop Relat Res* 2009b;467:638-44.

Clohisy JC, St John LC, Schutz AL. Surgical treatment of femoroacetabular impingement: a systematic review of the literature. *Clin Orthop Relat Res* 2010;468:555-64.

Colvin AC, Harrast J, Harner C. Trends in hip arthroscopy. *J Bone Joint Surg Am* 2012;94:e23.

Dolan MM, Heyworth BE, Bedi A, Duke G, Kelly BT. CT reveals a high incidence of osseous abnormalities in hips with labral tears. *Clin Orthop Relat Res* 2011;469:831-8.

Domb BG, Stake CE, Botser IB, Jackson TJ. Surgical dislocation of the hip versus arthroscopic treatment of femoroacetabular impingement: a prospective matched-pair study with average 2-year follow-up. *Arthroscopy* 2013;29:1506-13.

Dunn DM. Anteversion of the neck of the femur; a method of measurement. J *Bone Joint Surg Br* 1952;34-B:181-6.

Duthon VB, Charbonnier C, Kolo FC, et al. Correlation of clinical and magnetic resonance imaging findings in hips of elite female ballet dancers. *Arthroscopy* 2013;29:411-9.

Eijer H, Myers SR, Ganz R. Anterior femoroacetabular impingement after femoral neck fractures. *J Orthop Trauma* 2001;15:475-81.

Emara K, Samir W, Motasem eH, Ghafar KA. Conservative treatment for mild femoroacetabular impingement. *J Orthop Surg (Hong Kong)* 2011;19:41-5.

Epstein NJ, Safran MR. Stress fracture of the acetabular rim: arthroscopic reduction and internal fixation. A case report. *J Bone Joint Surg Am* 2009;91:1480-6.

Espinosa N, Rothenfluh DA, Beck M, Ganz R, Leunig M. Treatment of femoro-acetabular impingement: preliminary results of labral refixation. J *Bone Joint Surg Am* 2006;88:925-35.

Fowler J, Owens BD. Abdominal compartment syndrome after hip arthroscopy. *Arthroscopy* 2010;26:128-30.

Galbraith RT, Gelberman RH, Hajek PC, et al. Obesity and decreased femoral anteversion in adolescence. *J Orthop Res* 1987;5:523-8.

Ganz R, Gill TJ, Gautier E, Ganz K, Kr,gel N, Berlemann U. Surgical dislocation of the adult hip a technique with full access to the femoral head and acetabulum without the risk of avascular necrosis. *J Bone Joint Surg Br* 2001;83:1119-24.

Ganz R, Leunig M, Leunig-Ganz K, Harris WH. The etiology of osteoarthritis of the hip: an integrated mechanical concept. *Clin Orthop Relat Res* 2008;466:264-72.

Ganz R, Parvizi J, Beck M, Leunig M, N^tzli H, Siebenrock KA. Femoroacetabular impingement: a cause for osteoarthritis of the hip. *Clin Orthop Relat Res* 2003:112-20.

Gautier E, Ganz K, Kr‚gel N, Gill T, Ganz R. Anatomy of the medial femoral circumflex artery and its surgical implications. *J Bone Joint Surg Br* 2000;82:679-83.

Gerhardt MB, Romero AA, Silvers HJ, Harris DJ, Watanabe D, Mandelbaum BR. The prevalence of radiographic hip abnormalities in elite soccer players. *Am J Sports Med* 2012;40:584-8.

Geyer MR, Philippon MJ, Fagrelius TS, Briggs KK. Acetabular labral reconstruction with an iliotibial band autograft: outcome and survivorship analysis at minimum 3-year follow-up. *Am J Sports Med* 2013;41:1750-6.

Giles AE, Corneman NA, Bhachu S, et al. Shared morphology of slipped capital femoral epiphysis and femoroacetabular impingement in early-onset arthritis. *Orthopedics* 2013;36:e1365-70.

Goodman DA, Feighan JE, Smith AD, Latimer B, Buly RL, Cooperman DR. Subclinical slipped capital femoral epiphysis. Relationship to osteoarthrosis of the hip. *J Bone Joint Surg Am* 1997;79:1489-97.

Gosvig KK, Jacobsen S, Palm H, Sonne-Holm S, Magnusson E. A new radiological index for assessing asphericity of the femoral head in cam impingement. *J Bone Joint Surg Br* 2007;89:1309-16.

Gosvig KK, Jacobsen S, Sonne-Holm S, Gebuhr P. The prevalence of cam-type deformity of the hip joint: a survey of 4151 subjects of the Copenhagen Osteoarthritis Study. *Acta Radiol* 2008;49:436-41.

Grabinski R, Ou D, Saunder K, et al. Protocol for CT in the position of discomfort: Preoperative assessment of femoroacetabular impingement - how we do it and what the surgeon wants to know. *J Med Imaging Radiat Oncol* 2014.

Hack K, Di Primio G, Rakhra K, Beaulé PE. Prevalence of cam-type femoroacetabular impingement morphology in asymptomatic volunteers. *J Bone Joint Surg Am* 2010;92:2436-44.

Haddad B, Konan S, Haddad FS. Debridement versus re-attachment of acetabular labral tears: A review of the literature and quantitative analysis. *Bone Joint J* 2014;96-B:24-30.

Hammoud S, Bedi A, Magennis E, Meyers WC, Kelly BT. High incidence of athletic pubalgia symptoms in professional athletes with symptomatic femoroacetabular impingement. *Arthroscopy* 2012;28:1388-95.

Harris JD, McCormick FM, Abrams GD, et al. Complications and reoperations during and after hip arthroscopy: a systematic review of 92 studies and more than 6,000 patients. *Arthroscopy* 2013;29:589-95.

Hergan K, Oser W, Moriggl B. Acetabular ossicles: normal variant or disease entity? *Eur Radiol* 2000;10:624-8.

Hunt D, Prather H, Harris Hayes M, Clohisy JC. Clinical outcomes analysis of conservative and surgical treatment of patients with clinical indications of prearthritic, intra-articular hip disorders. *PM R* 2012;4:479-87.

Ito K, Minka MA, Leunig M, Werlen S, Ganz R. Femoroacetabular impingement and the cam-effect. A MRI-based quantitative anatomical study of the femoral head-neck offset. *J Bone Joint Surg Br* 2001;83:171-6.

Jaberi FM, Parvizi J. Hip pain in young adults: femoroacetabular impingement. *J Arthroplasty* 2007;22:37-42.

Jackson TJ, Stake CE, Stone JC, Lindner D, El Bitar YF, Domb BG. Radiographic, histologic, and arthroscopic findings in amorphous calcifications of the hip labrum. *Arthroscopy* 2014;30:456-61.

Jamali AA, Mladenov K, Meyer DC, et al. Anteroposterior pelvic radiographs to assess acetabular retroversion: high validity of the "cross-over-sign". *J Orthop Res* 2007;25:758-65.

Johnson AC, Shaman MA, Ryan TG. Femoroacetabular impingement in former high-level youth soccer players. *Am J Sports Med* 2012;40:1342-6.

Kalberer F, Sierra RJ, Madan SS, Ganz R, Leunig M. Ischial spine projection into the pelvis: a new sign for acetabular retroversion. *Clin Orthop Relat Res* 2008;466:677-83.

Kang AC, Gooding AJ, Coates MH, Goh TD, Armour P, Rietveld J. Computed tomography assessment of hip joints in asymptomatic individuals in relation to femoroacetabular impingement. *Am J Sports Med* 2010;38:1160-5.

Kapron AL, Anderson AE, Aoki SK, et al. Radiographic prevalence of femoroacetabular impingement in collegiate football players: AAOS Exhibit Selection. *J Bone Joint Surg Am* 2011;93:e111(1-10).

Karthikeyan S, Roberts S, Griffin D. Microfracture for acetabular chondral defects in patients with femoroacetabular impingement: results at second-look arthroscopic surgery. *Am J Sports Med* 2012;40:2725-30.

Kim YT, Azuma H. The nerve endings of the acetabular labrum. *Clin Orthop Relat Res* 1995:176-81.

Klit J, Gosvig K, Magnussen E, et al. Cam deformity and hip degeneration are common after fixation of a slipped capital femoral epiphysis. *Acta Orthop* 2014:1-7.

Kolo FC, Charbonnier C, Pfirrmann CW, et al. Extreme hip motion in professional ballet dancers: dynamic and morphological evaluation based on magnetic resonance imaging. *Skeletal Radiol* 2013;42:689-98.

Konan S, Rayan F, Haddad FS. Is the frog lateral plain radiograph a reliable predictor of the alpha angle in femoroacetabular impingement? *J Bone Joint Surg Br* 2010;92:47-50.

Kubo T, Horii M, Harada Y, et al. Radial-sequence magnetic resonance imaging in evaluation of acetabular labrum. *J Orthop Sci* 1999;4:328-32.

Laage H, Barnett JC, Brady JM, et al. Horizontal lateral roentgenography of the hip in children; a preliminary report. *J Bone Joint Surg Am* 1953;35-A:387-98.

Laborie LB, Lehmann TG, EngesÊter I, Eastwood DM, EngesÊter LB, Rosendahl K. Prevalence of radiographic findings thought to be associated with femoroacetabular impingement in a population-based cohort of 2081 healthy young adults. *Radiology* 2011;260:494-502.

Lahner M, von Schulze Pellengahr C, Walter PA, et al. Biomechanical and functional indicators in male semiprofessional soccer players with increased hip alpha angles vs. amateur soccer players. *BMC Musculoskelet Disord* 2014a;15:88.

Lahner M, Walter PA, von Schulze Pellengahr C, Hagen M, von Engelhardt LV, Lukas C. Comparative study of the femoroacetabular impingement (FAI) prevalence in male semiprofessional and amateur soccer players. *Arch Orthop Trauma Surg* 2014b;134:1135-41.

Larson CM, Giveans MR, Stone RM. Arthroscopic debridement versus refixation of the acetabular labrum associated with femoroacetabular impingement: mean 3.5-year follow-up. *Am J Sports Med* 2012;40:1015-21.

Larson CM, Sikka RS, Sardelli MC, et al. Increasing alpha angle is predictive of athletic-related "hip" and "groin" pain in collegiate National Football League prospects. *Arthroscopy* 2013;29:405-10.

Larson CM, Stone RM. The rarely encountered rim fracture that contributes to both femoroacetabular impingement and hip stability: a report of 2 cases of arthroscopic partial excision and internal fixation. *Arthroscopy* 2011;27:1018-22.

Leunig M, Beck M, Kalhor M, Kim YJ, Werlen S, Ganz R. Fibrocystic changes at anterosuperior femoral neck: prevalence in hips with femoroacetabular impingement. *Radiology* 2005;236:237-46.

Lovett Carter D, Kennedy N. What Are Athletes' Perceptions of Rehabilitation Outcome One Year Post Hip Arthroscopy? *J Sport Rehabil* 2013.

Mamisch TC, Bittersohl B, Hughes T, et al. Magnetic resonance imaging of the hip at 3 Tesla: clinical value in femoroacetabular impingement of the hip and current concepts. *Semin Musculoskelet Radiol* 2008;12:212-22.

Martinez AE, Li SM, Ganz R, Beck M. Os acetabuli in femoro-acetabular impingement: stress fracture or unfused secondary ossification centre of the acetabular rim? *Hip Int* 2006;16:281-6.

Matsuda DK, Hanami D. Hip arthroscopy for challenging deformities: posterior cam decompression. *Arthrosc Tech* 2013;2:e45-9.

McDonald JE, Herzog MM, Philippon MJ. Return to play after hip arthroscopy with microfracture in elite athletes. *Arthroscopy* 2013;29:330-5.

McDonald JE, Herzog MM, Philippon MJ. Performance outcomes in professional hockey players following arthroscopic treatment of FAI and microfracture of the hip. *Knee Surg Sports Traumatol Arthrosc* 2014;22:915-9.

Mei-Dan O, McConkey MO, Brick M. Catastrophic failure of hip arthroscopy due to iatrogenic instability: can partial division of the ligamentum teres and iliofemoral ligament cause subluxation? *Arthroscopy* 2012;28:440-5.

Meyer DC, Beck M, Ellis T, Ganz R, Leunig M. Comparison of six radiographic projections to assess femoral head/neck asphericity. *Clin Orthop Relat Res* 2006;445:181-5.

Milone MT, Bedi A, Poultsides L, et al. Novel CT-based three-dimensional software improves the characterization of cam morphology. *Clin Orthop Relat Res* 2013;471:2484-91.

Mose K. Methods of measuring in Legg-CalvÈ-Perthes disease with special regard to the prognosis. *Clin Orthop Relat Res* 1980:103-9.

Murray RO, Duncan C. Athletic activity in adolescence as an etiological factor in degenerative hip disease. *J Bone Joint Surg Br* 1971;53:406-19.

Myers SR, Eijer H, Ganz R. Anterior femoroacetabular impingement after periacetabular osteotomy. *Clin Orthop Relat Res* 1999:93-9.

Naal FD, Miozzari HH, Sch‰r M, Hesper T, N˜tzli HP. Midterm results of surgical hip dislocation for the treatment of femoroacetabular impingement. *Am J Sports Med* 2012;40:1501-10.

Naal FD, Miozzari HH, Wyss TF, N˜tzli HP. Surgical hip dislocation for the treatment of femoroacetabular impingement in high-level athletes. *Am J Sports Med* 2011;39:544-50.

Nasreddine AY, Heyworth BE, Zurakowski D, Kocher MS. A reduction in body mass index lowers risk for bilateral slipped capital femoral epiphysis. *Clin Orthop Relat Res* 2013;471:2137-44.

Nepple JJ, Brophy RH, Matava MJ, Wright RW, Clohisy JC. Radiographic findings of femoroacetabular impingement in National Football League

Combine athletes undergoing radiographs for previous hip or groin pain. *Arthroscopy* 2012a;28:1396-403.

Nepple JJ, Byrd JW, Siebenrock KA, Prather H, Clohisy JC. Overview of treatment options, clinical results, and controversies in the management of femoroacetabular impingement. *J Am Acad Orthop Surg* 2013;21 Suppl 1:S53-8.

Nepple JJ, Martel JM, Kim YJ, Zaltz I, Clohisy JC, Group AS. Do plain radiographs correlate with CT for imaging of cam-type femoroacetabular impingement? *Clin Orthop Relat Res* 2012b;470:3313-20.

Ng VY, Ellis TJ. More than just a bump: cam-type femoroacetabular impingement and the evolution of the femoral neck. *Hip Int* 2011;21:1-8.

Nho SJ, Magennis EM, Singh CK, Kelly BT. Outcomes after the arthroscopic treatment of femoroacetabular impingement in a mixed group of high-level athletes. *Am J Sports Med* 2011;39 Suppl:14S-9S.

Nicholls AS, Kiran A, Pollard TC, et al. The association between hip morphology parameters and nineteen-year risk of end-stage osteoarthritis of the hip: a nested case-control study. *Arthritis Rheum* 2011;63:3392-400.

Nötzli HP, Wyss TF, Stoecklin CH, Schmid MR, Treiber K, Hodler J. The contour of the femoral head-neck junction as a predictor for the risk of anterior impingement. *J Bone Joint Surg Br* 2002;84:556-60.

Novais EN, Heyworth BE, Stamoulis C, Sullivan K, Millis MB, Kim YJ. Open surgical treatment of femoroacetabular impingement in adolescent athletes: preliminary report on improvement of physical activity level. *J Pediatr Orthop* 2014;34:287-94.

Panzer S, Augat P, Esch U. CT assessment of herniation pits: prevalence, characteristics, and potential association with morphological predictors of femoroacetabular impingement. *Eur Radiol* 2008;18:1869-75.

Park MS, Yoon SJ, Kim YJ, Chung WC. Hip arthroscopy for femoroacetabular impingement: the changing nature and severity of associated complications over time. *Arthroscopy* 2014;30:957-63.

Parvizi J, Bican O, Bender B, et al. Arthroscopy for labral tears in patients with developmental dysplasia of the hip: a cautionary note. *J Arthroplasty* 2009;24:110-3.

Peters CL, Erickson JA. Treatment of femoro-acetabular impingement with surgical dislocation and dÈbridement in young adults. *J Bone Joint Surg Am* 2006;88:1735-41.

Peters CL, Schabel K, Anderson L, Erickson J. Open treatment of femoroacetabular impingement is associated with clinical improvement and low complication rate at short-term followup. *Clin Orthop Relat Res* 2010;468:504-10.

Pfirrmann CW, Duc SR, Zanetti M, Dora C, Hodler J. MR arthrography of acetabular cartilage delamination in femoroacetabular cam impingement. *Radiology* 2008;249:236-41.

Philippon MJ, Briggs KK, Carlisle JC, Patterson DC. Joint space predicts THA after hip arthroscopy in patients 50 years and older. *Clin Orthop Relat Res* 2013a;471:2492-6.

Philippon MJ, Ho CP, Briggs KK, Stull J, LaPrade RF. Prevalence of increased alpha angles as a measure of cam-type femoroacetabular impingement in youth ice hockey players. *Am J Sports Med* 2013b;41:1357-62.

Philippon MJ, Maxwell RB, Johnston TL, Schenker M, Briggs KK. Clinical presentation of femoroacetabular impingement. *Knee Surg Sports Traumatol Arthrosc* 2007;15:1041-7.

Philippon MJ, Schenker ML, Briggs KK, Maxwell RB. Can microfracture produce repair tissue in acetabular chondral defects? *Arthroscopy* 2008;24:46-50.

Rab GT. The geometry of slipped capital femoral epiphysis: implications for movement, impingement, and corrective osteotomy. *J Pediatr Orthop* 1999;19:419-24.

Rakhra KS, Sheikh AM, Allen D, BeaulÈ PE. Comparison of MRI alpha angle measurement planes in femoroacetabular impingement. *Clin Orthop Relat Res* 2009;467:660-5.

Reichenbach S, J,ni P, Werlen S, et al. Prevalence of cam-type deformity on hip magnetic resonance imaging in young males: a cross-sectional study. *Arthritis Care Res* (Hoboken) 2010;62:1319-27

Riley GM, McWalter EJ, Stevens KJ, Safran MR, Lattanzi R, Gold GE. MRI of the Hip for the evaluation of femoroacetabular impingement; past, present, and future. *J Magn Reson Imaging* 2014.

Ross JR, Bedi A, Stone RM, et al. Intraoperative Fluoroscopic Imaging to Treat Cam Deformities: Correlation With 3-Dimensional Computed Tomography. *Am J Sports Med* 2014;42:1370-6.

Sampson TG. Complications of hip arthroscopy. *Clin Sports Med* 2001;20:831-5.

Sarkar JS, Haddad FS, Crean SV, Brooks P. Acute calcific tendinitis of the rectus femoris. *J Bone Joint Surg Br* 1996;78:814-6.

Schaberg JE, Harper MC, Allen WC. The snapping hip syndrome. *Am J Sports Med* 1984;12:361-5.

Schilders E, Dimitrakopoulou A, Bismil Q, Marchant P, Cooke C. Arthroscopic treatment of labral tears in femoroacetabular impingement: a comparative study of refixation and resection with a minimum two-year follow-up. *J Bone Joint Surg Br* 2011;93:1027-32.

Schmitz MR, Campbell SE, Fajardo RS, Kadrmas WR. Identification of acetabular labral pathological changes in asymptomatic volunteers using optimized, noncontrast 1.5-T magnetic resonance imaging. *Am J Sports Med* 2012;40:1337-41.

Siebenrock KA, Behning A, Mamisch TC, Schwab JM. Growth plate alteration precedes cam-type deformity in elite basketball players. *Clin Orthop Relat Res* 2013a;471:1084-91.

Siebenrock KA, Ferner F, Noble PC, Santore RF, Werlen S, Mamisch TC. The cam-type deformity of the proximal femur arises in childhood in response to vigorous sporting activity. *Clin Orthop Relat Res* 2011;469:3229-40.

Siebenrock KA, Kalbermatten DF, Ganz R. Effect of pelvic tilt on acetabular retroversion: a study of pelves from cadavers. *Clin Orthop Relat Res* 2003:241-8.

Siebenrock KA, Kaschka I, Frauchiger L, Werlen S, Schwab JM. Prevalence of cam-type deformity and hip pain in elite ice hockey players before and after the end of growth. *Am J Sports Med* 2013b;41:2308-13.

Siebenrock KA, Kienle KP, Steppacher SD, Tannast M, Mamisch TC, von Rechenberg B. Biochemical MRI Predicts Hip Osteoarthritis in an Experimental Ovine Femoroacetabular Impingement Model. *Clin Orthop Relat Res* 2014.

Siebenrock KA, Schoeniger R, Ganz R. Anterior femoro-acetabular impingement due to acetabular retroversion. Treatment with periacetabular osteotomy. *J Bone Joint Surg Am* 2003;85-A:278-86.

Sierra RJ. The management of acetabular retroversion with reverse periacetabular osteotomy. *Instr Course Lect* 2013;62:305-13.

Singh PJ, O'Donnell JM. The outcome of hip arthroscopy in Australian football league players: a review of 27 hips. *Arthroscopy* 2010;26:743-9.

Sink EL, BeaulÈ PE, Sucato D, et al. Multicenter study of complications following surgical dislocation of the hip. *J Bone Joint Surg Am* 2011;93:1132-6.

Smith TO, Hilton G, Toms AP, Donell ST, Hing CB. The diagnostic accuracy of acetabular labral tears using magnetic resonance imaging and magnetic resonance arthrography: a meta-analysis. *Eur Radiol* 2011;21:863-74.

Smith-Petersen MN. The classic: Treatment of malum coxae senilis, old slipped upper femoral epiphysis, intrapelvic protrusion of the acetabulum, and coxa plana by means of acetabuloplasty. 1936. *Clin Orthop Relat Res* 2009;467:608-15.

Stafford GH, Bunn JR, Villar RN. Arthroscopic repair of delaminated acetabular articular cartilage using fibrin adhesive. Results at one to three years. *Hip Int* 2011;21:744-50.

Steppacher SD, Huemmer C, Schwab JM, Tannast M, Siebenrock KA. Surgical hip dislocation for treatment of femoroacetabular impingement: factors predicting 5-year survivorship. *Clin Orthop Relat Res* 2014;472:337-48.

Stulberg SD, Cordell LD, Harris WH, Ramsey PL, MacEwen GD. Unrecognised childhood hip disease: a major cause of idiopathic osteoarthritis of the hip. *Proceedings of the Third Open Scientific Meeting of the Hip Society. St Louis (MO): Mosby;* 1975. p. 212–8.

Stull JD, Philippon MJ, LaPrade RF. "At-risk" positioning and hip biomechanics of the Peewee ice hockey sprint start. *Am J Sports Med* 2011;39 Suppl:29S-35S.

Sundberg TP, Toomayan GA, Major NM. Evaluation of the acetabular labrum at 3.0-T MR imaging compared with 1.5-T MR arthrography: preliminary experience. *Radiology* 2006;238:706-11.

Sutter R, Zubler V, Hoffmann A, et al. Hip MRI: how useful is intraarticular contrast material for evaluating surgically proven lesions of the labrum and articular cartilage? *AJR Am J Roentgenol* 2014;202:160-9.

Tannast M, Goricki D, Beck M, Murphy SB, Siebenrock KA. Hip damage occurs at the zone of femoroacetabular impingement. *Clin Orthop Relat Res* 2008;466:273-80.

Toomayan GA, Holman WR, Major NM, Kozlowicz SM, Vail TP. Sensitivity of MR arthrography in the evaluation of acetabular labral tears. *AJR Am J Roentgenol* 2006;186:449-53.

Tönnis D. Congenital Dysplasia and Dislocation of the Hip in Children and Adults. Berlin, Germany, New York, NY: *Springer;* 1987

Tveit M, Rosengren BE, Nilsson J, Karlsson MK. Former male elite athletes have a higher prevalence of osteoarthritis and arthroplasty in the hip and knee than expected. *Am J Sports Med* 2012;40:527-33.

Van Thiel GS, Harris JD, Kang RW, et al. Age-related differences in radiographic parameters for femoroacetabular impingement in hip arthroplasty patients. *Arthroscopy* 2013;29:1182-7.

Vingård E, Alfredsson L, Goldie I, Hogstedt C. Sports and osteoarthrosis of the hip. An epidemiologic study. *Am J Sports Med* 1993;21:195-200.

Vingård E, Alfredsson L, Malchau H. Osteoarthrosis of the hip in women and its relationship to physical load from sports activities. *Am J Sports Med* 1998;26:78-82.

Wahoff M, Ryan M. Rehabilitation after hip femoroacetabular impingement arthroscopy. *Clin Sports Med* 2011;30:463-82.

Wall PD, Fernandez M, Griffin DR, Foster NE. Nonoperative treatment for femoroacetabular impingement: a systematic review of the literature. *PM R 2013;5:418-26.*

Wenger DE, Kendell KR, Miner MR, Trousdale RT. Acetabular labral tears rarely occur in the absence of bony abnormalities. *Clin Orthop Relat Res* 2004:145-50.

Wensaas A, Gunderson RB, Svenningsen S, Terjesen T. Femoroacetabular impingement after slipped upper femoral epiphysis: the radiological diagnosis and clinical outcome at long-term follow-up. *J Bone Joint Surg Br* 2012;94:1487-93.

Wiberg G. Shelf operation in congenital dysplasia of the acetabulum and in subluxation and dislocation of the hip. *J Bone Joint Surg Am* 1953;35-A:65-80.

Wijdicks CA, Philippon MJ, Civitarese DM, LaPrade RF. A mandated change in goalie pad width has no effect on ice hockey goaltender hip kinematics. *Clin J Sport Med* 2014;24:403-8.

Yasunaga Y, Ikuta Y, Kanazawa T, Takahashi K, Hisatome T. The state of the articular cartilage at the time of surgery as an indication for rotational acetabular osteotomy. *J Bone Joint Surg Br* 2001;83:1001-4.

Zaltz I, Kelly BT, Hetsroni I, Bedi A. The crossover sign overestimates acetabular retroversion. *Clin Orthop Relat Res* 2013;471:2463-70.

Zlatkin MB, Pevsner D, Sanders TG, Hancock CR, Ceballos CE, Herrera MF. Acetabular labral tears and cartilage lesions of the hip: indirect MR arthrographic correlation with arthroscopy--a preliminary study. *AJR Am J Roentgenol* 2010;194:709-14.

In: Sports Injuries
Editor: Gabrielle Hopkins

ISBN: 978-1-63463-305-5

Chapter 2

A SUMMARY OF CENTRAL NERVOUS SYSTEM INJURIES ASSOCIATED WITH THE SPORT OF ICE HOCKEY

***Ozan Toy*[*1], *Arielle Berkowitz*[2], *Ronald Bogdasarian*[3] *and Mill Etienne*[4]**
Thc Commonwealth Medical College
[1] The Commonwealth Medical College, Scranton, PA, US
[2] Good Samaritan Hospital, Suffern, NY, US
[3] The Commonwealth Medical College, Scranton, PA, US
[4] New York Medical College, Valhalla, NY, US

ABSTRACT

Objective: To determine the types of injuries affecting the Central Nervous System (CNS) throughout the history of ice hockey and the estimated incidence of each type of CNS injury based on the literature.

Background: Ice hockey is a contact sport characterized by high acceleration and deceleration forces, fast skating and puck velocities, body checking and forceful stick use. Athletes can receive impacts from opposing players, the boards, pucks, sticks, and goal posts. These aspects of ice hockey pose risks for injury to the brain and spinal cord.

* Correspondence concerning this article should be addressed to Ozan Toy, 10 Wilton Dr., Allendale, NJ 07401. E-mail: otoy@wesleyan.edu.

Identifying CNS injuries and associated incidence in ice hockey will help clinicians to better inform participating athletes.

Methods: We conducted a literature search via Pubmed. Additionally, we utilized Google and Wikipedia to find media reports regarding CNS injuries in ice hockey. We used the following search terms: hockey concussion, hockey second impact syndrome, hockey spinal cord injury, hockey paralysis, hockey head trauma, hockey death.

Results & Conclusion: The following CNS injuries were the most common: Concussion (0.2 to 6.6 per 1000 player hours) and Spinal Cord Injury (5 per 1000 player hours). Other rare injuries of undetermined incidence include: Second Impact Syndrome, Subarachnoid Hemorrhage, Subdural Hematoma, Epidural Hematoma, Spinal Cord Concussion, and Vertebral Hemorrhage. Controversial associations with long term consequences of head impact in ice hockey include Post-Concussive Syndrome and Chronic Traumatic Encephalopathy (CTE). It is our recommendation that all ice hockey players, their parents, and healthcare professionals are informed of the risks of the game.

INTRODUCTION

In the United States, there are currently over 500,000 registered ice hockey players (USA Hockey). The concussion epidemic and discovery of chronic traumatic encephalopathy in National Hockey League (NHL) players has led to growing fears regarding risks to neurological health in the sport of ice hockey.

Players are at risk for CNS injury due to the nature of the sport. Ice hockey is characterized by high acceleration and deceleration forces, fast skating and puck velocities, body checking and forceful stick use. Additionally, athletes can receive impacts from opposing players, the boards, pucks, sticks, and goal posts. Nearly all levels of competition have attempted to reduce incidence of injury via rule changes, more stringent penalties, and mandatory protective equipment. However, the efficacy of such measures is not known. Hockey players can attain skating speeds of nearly 30 miles per hour and some players can shoot a puck over 100 mph.

We reviewed substantial literature describing central nervous system injuries such as concussion, spinal cord injury, subdural hematoma, subarachnoid hemorrhage, epidural hematoma, spinal cord concussion, and vertebral hemorrhage. To our knowledge, this is the most recent and complete review of CNS injuries associated with the sport of ice hockey.

METHODS

We conducted a literature search via Pubmed. Additionally, we utilized Wikipedia and Google to find media reports regarding CNS injuries in ice hockey. We used the following search terms: hockey concussion, hockey spinal cord Injury, hockey paralysis, Hockey head trauma, hockey death.

CONCUSSION

Concussions are the most common injury affecting the CNS in ice hockey. Honey's review indicated children aged 5 to 14 experiencing concussions at a rate of 2.8 per 1000 player-hours and high school players at 2.7 concussions per 100 player hours. Additionally Honey cited another study of elite amateurs as high as 6.6 per 1000 players hours (Honey 43-46). Benson et al. reported of 559 regular season concussions suffered by NHL players over the course of seven years. The mean number of total concussions per year was 80, with a rate of 5.8 concussions per 100 players per season. The estimated incidence density was 1.8 concussions per 1000 game player-hours (Benson et al. 905-911). Finally, one study on concussion incidence at the professional level over the 3 seasons analyzed revealed 5.23 concussions per 100 NHL regular season games and 5.05 concussions per 100 OHL regular season games (IRR 1.04; 95% CI 1.01, 1.50). When injuries described as concussion-like or suspicious of concussion were included, incidences rose to 8.8 and 7.1 per 100 games respectively (IRR 1.23; 95% CI 0.81, 1.32), Donaldson, Asbridge, and Cusimano.

Gerberich, in an epidemiological study of ice hockey players, discovered that 9% of the 251 athletes experienced a concussion (loss of consciousness orawareness), accounting for 12% of the total number of injuries. 27% of concussed players had experienced a prior loss of consciousness. The risk of concussion increased 4.1% for students who reported playing ice hockey in order to release aggression and tension. 22.5% of head injuries were sustained during high velocity breakout plays. The main cause of injuries were collisions with another player (34%), the boards (19.8%), or the frame of the net (19.8%). 89% of players felt that face masks aided their safety, while 2% felt that it put them at higher risk of injury. Players who reported inadequate vision due to face masks were two times more likely to be injured and five times more likely to experience a concussion (Gerberich et al. 59-64).

SPINAL CORD INJURY

Data was gathered from 42 ice hockey players in a study by Tator and Edmonds, ranging from 11 to 45 years old. Injuries to the spine were sustained during neck flexion (n=21), extension (n=6), and neutral placement (n=3). Although neck positioning was unknown for 12 of the players, in no case was there harm due to a direct blow. The most common site of injury was to the C5 vertebrae (n=9), C5-C6 region (n=9) resulting in fractures, including burst fractures, and/or dislocations (n=27). The majority of players (n=16) sustained incomplete motor/sensory loss (Tator and Edmonds 875-880).

Tator et al. examined spinal cord injuries resulting from ice hockey in Canada from 1943- 1999. A questionnaire was distributed to physicians and surgeons throughout Canada to compile data on spinal injuries in ice hockey since 1981. The authors included any injuries with thecriteria "defined as a fracture or dislocation of the spine with or without injury to the spinal cord or nerve roots, with or without a permanent neurologic deficit. Minor spinal injuries such as strains, sprains or whiplash were excluded." Findings revealed that among the 255 documented ice hockey injuries, 125 occurred among individuals ages 16-20. The majority of collisions resulted from being pushed or checked from behind (n=74), and most occurred by colliding with the boards (n=148). The precise location was given for 235 of the reported injuries with 83.5% of the injuries occurring at the level of the cervical vertebrae, 5.1% were thoracic (T1-T11), 5.9% thoraco-lumbar (T11/12-L1/2) and 5.5% lumbo-sacral (L2-S5). Consequently, 75% of players sustained neurological deficits and 47.3% sustained a permanent injury. Injured players were classified as having complete motor and complete sensory loss, complete motor and incomplete sensory loss or complete motor loss only. Again, impact of the head with the boards after being checked or pushed from behind was the most common mechanism of spinal cord injury (Tator et al. 460-466).

The NCAA reported that from 2001-2002, spinal injuries accounted for 9% of hockey injuries. The NCAA found that the most common site of fracture or dislocation was the C5-C7 region of the vertebral column. These injuries also most often occurred due to checks from behind. According to the "Canadian ThinkFirst-SportSmart Sports and Recreational Injuries Research and Prevention Center Registry, an average of 17 cases of spinal injuries per year occurred, peaking in 1995 with 26 injuries " (Boden and Jarvis 55-68, vii).

SECOND IMPACT SYNDROME

While Second impact syndrome is considered a rare occurrence, it is a recognized complication of multiple concussions. Our review of the literature found one case of a 16 year old hockey player that died following a probable diagnosis SIS after meeting criteria (b), (c), and (d) established for the diagnosis of SIS. The following criteria were used to make the diagnosis of SIS: "(a) Medical review after a witnessed first concussion. (b) Documentation of ongoing symptoms following the first impact up to the time of the second impact. (c) Witnessed second head impact with a subsequent rapid cerebral deterioration. (d) Neuropathologic or neuroimaging evidence of cerebral swelling without significant intracranial hematoma or cause for edema."

According to McCrory and Berkovic , in 1968 a 16 year old hockey player struck the back of his head on the ice and experienced a brief loss of consciousness. Witnesses confirmed this event. After the initial head trauma, the ice hockey player experienced symptoms of headache and unsteadiness. Approximately four days after the first head trauma, the ice hockey player resumed athletic activity. Unfortunately, he suffered another heavy body check, striking his left temporal bone on the ice. Again, he experienced loss of consciousness. Within two hours of this second impact, the ice hockey player died. On pathology report, subarachnoid hemorrhage, small subdural hematoma, occipital contusion, and cerebral edema were noted.

SELECTED CASE REPORTS OF CNS INJURIES

Spinal Cord Concussion

Spinal cord concussion (SCC) is an unusual injury that can result in a transient quadriplegia. The predominant cause of SCC is spinal stenosis, but a search of the literature revealed a case in a 33 year old professional ice hockey player who developed this condition after a blow by an ice hockey puck in the upper cervical region.

This ice hockey player was positioned with his back facing the opposing team's goal. Subsequently, the player was checked from behind and fell forward. As the player was falling forward, a puck was shot at high speed towards him. The player flexed his neck to avoid the puck from hitting his face. In doing so, he exposed the dorsum of his neck was struck by the puck in his upper cervical region. His left shoulder and the left side of his head were the first body parts to make contact with the ice. At the time of being struck with the puck, the patient experienced significant neck pain and was unable to feel or move below his neck. While being assessed on the ice, he regained some uncoordinated movements with a sensation of "pins and needles" throughout his body. During transportation to the hospital, the patient regained normal movement and sensation nearly 30 minutes after the injury. During medical evaluation in the ER, the patient demonstrated no neurological abnormalities, with tenderness and bruising in the cervical region. The patient was followed up by team physicians at 2 weeks and 6 weeks post-injury. Medical evaluations demonstrated no neurological abnormalities or symptoms. At 6 weeks, the patient demonstrated full cervical range of motion and minor tenderness over the C3 Vertebrae. Subsequently, the patient was cleared to resume athletic activities (Winder, Brett, and Hurlbert 677-680).

This case report is unique in that the patient lacked any spinal canal stenosis. Rather, he experienced SCC due to a large focal force which resulted in soft tissue swelling and fracture of a spinous process. The average velocity of an ice hockey puck shot at the professional level is 90 mph, or 145 km/hr. The weight of an ice hockey puck is 170 grams. The kinetic energy ($Joules = \frac{1}{2} Mass \times Velocity^2$) of a fired ice hockey puck often reaches 140 Joules. The authors, Winder, Brett and Hurlbert suggest this impact likely caused soft tissue injury and, indirectly, transfers kinetic injury to the spinal cord causing SCC. The authors also suggest that the impact of the puck caused a sudden acceleration of the spinal canal and cord, countered by an equally sudden deceleration as the spinal cord exceeded its cerebrospinal fluid buffer leading to impaction of the spinal canal over several spinal segments. This mechanism is termed the "water-hammer" effect. Regardless, the authors concluded that one or both of these mechanisms may have caused a widespread change in local ion permeability at the C-3 level, resulting in transient quadriplegia.

Post-Concussive Syndrome and Chronic Traumatic Encephalopathy

The Center for the Study of Traumatic Encephalopathy (CSTE) at Boston University School of Medicine performed post-mortem analysis of the brains and spinal cords of athletes and military veterans exposed to repetitive mild traumatic brain injury. Each subject's brain trauma history, substance abuse history, athletic history and cognitive and behavioral profiles, among other matters, were queried via post-mortem interviews with next of kin. These interviews were performed by a neuropsychologist, blind to neuropathological results. Next of kin were also blind to results of neuropathological assessment. 85 Brains from individuals exposed to repetitive head trauma were compared with 18 cognitively normal age and gender-matched control subjects for signs of p-tau protein pathology. Controls had no known history of contact sports or mild traumatic brain injury. Diagnosis of CTE was defined by "perivascular foci of p-tau immunoreactive astrocytic tangles and neurofibrillary tangles; (ii) irregular cortical distribution of p-tau immunoreactive neurofibrillary tangles and astrocytic tangles with a predilection for the depth of cerebral sulci; (iii) clusters of subpial and periventricular astrocytic tangles in the cerebral cortex, diencephalon, basal ganglia and brainstem; and (iv) neurofibrillary tangles in the cerebral cortex located preferentially in the superficial layers" (McKee et al. 43-64).

A total of 8 subjects from the group of 85 examined for chronic traumatic encephalopathy had a history of playing ice hockey. Out of the total of eight athletes with a history of playing both professional and amateur ice hockey, five demonstrated a presence of CTE on examination. Only one case of CTE was found in an amateur ice hockey player, but this athlete's brain was analyzed at an advanced age and evidence of Alzheimers and Parkinsons was demonstrated.

The validity of a CTE diagnosis is questionable due to confounding variability with other dementias. Moreover, of the five former professional hockey players undergoing neuropathological analysis, four showed signs of CTE. Playing professional hockey was significantly associated with the development of CTE (Odds Ratio=8). Only one professional player did not have CTE. This was the youngest athlete of the group at20 years old. He did not play in the NHL, but rather in another professional league.

It should be mentioned that the majority of the ice hockey players' brains donated to this study belonged to players with repetitive brain injuries. Their specimens may over-estimate the brain trauma in an average ice hockey player. That said, participating in the NHL was significantly associated with development of CTE (Odds Ratio = 21). Every NHL player analyzed had CTE. Three of the four former NHL players had stage II CTE, one had stage III CTE and Lewy body disease (mean age 51.3 years, range 28–73 years). However, only three of the four were symptomatic at the time of death.

The NHL is considered the most physically demanding ice hockey league. It is not surprising that playing in this league was identified as a significant risk factor. Conversely, age below 29 years, is associated with decreased findings of CTE (Odds Ratio: 1/8). Only one player demonstrated CTE below the age of 29. This player was an enforcer with a significant history of fighting throughout his entire, albeit short, career (ESPN, 2011). The presence of CTE at a young age due to participation in the sport of ice hockey is less likely than the presence of CTE in a retired hockey player with accumulated head trauma.

Fatal Head and Neck Trauma

Sudden Death due to Neck Blows among Amateur Hockey Players

Maron performed a prospective cohort study which included autopsy on young athletes who succumbed to sudden death. He identified six male ice hockey players ages 9 to 30 years who died as a result of trauma to the neck from 1992 to 2002. Traumatic blows occurred as a result of a puck in 5 cases (n=5) and a fist during an altercation (n=1). Each collapsed immediately and resuscitative efforts were unsuccessful. Findings revealed that all of the athletes sustained blows to the lateral or posterolateral neck area—an exposed region adjacent to the helmet and neck guard. These blows resulted in dissected and ruptured vertebral arteries (n=4) and internal carotid arteries (n=1). The precise location of injury for one individual was unclear. Autopsies revealed rapid accumulation of blood within the basilar cistern, Sylvian fissures and ventricles, as well as brainstem herniation. Autopsies did not demonstrate evidence of an aneurysm in any case (Maron et al., 2003).

Blunt Carotid Artery Injury

Pretre presents a case report of damage to the carotid artery as a result of blunt trauma from a hockey stick to the neck sustained during an ice hockey match. The patient developed a traumatic pseudoaneurysm of the right common carotid artery, which subsequently embolized after a latency period of twenty days post- trauma. The patient presented with severe headache and developed a left hemisyndrome, altered level of consciousness, stupor and hemianopsy. Seven days after the ischemic episode, the patient expired. An autopsy was performed and demonstrated "A massive infarction of the right cerebral hemisphere, cerebral hypertension, and tentorial herniation along with pseudoaneurysm" (Pretre et al., year).

Fatal Traumatic Vertebral Artery Aneurysm Rupture

A 34-year-old hockey player struck over the left mastoid region by a puck suffered a fatal rupture of a left vertebral artery berry aneurysm. He became apneic within seconds of the injury and lacked any brainstem reflex within minutes. Computerized tomography scanning of his head revealed extensive subarachnoid hemorrhage and loss of cortical gray–white differentiation. He died later that day and an autopsy was performed. Postmortem examination showed massive subarachnoid hemorrhage in the posterior fossa and the remnants of a berry aneurysm near the origin of the left vertebral artery (Sahjpaul et al. 822-824).

Unspecified Fatal Head Trauma

A search of Google and Wikipedia provided media reports regarding amateur and professional ice hockey players that suffered from severe neurological injury and subsequent death.

According to the Ottawa Sun Newspaper, on March 7 1907, 22 year old Owen McCourt died the morning after a fight between two hockey teams. McCourt suffered a brain injury and was left unconscious. The article notes that a fracture of the skull was present and that upon operation there was "a broken blood vessel in the brain". It is believe that McCourt experienced blows from opposing players' hockey sticks ("Hockey Player Succumbs").

On January 15 1967, at the age of 29 as a member of the Minnesota Northstars, Bill Masterton became the only NHL player to die a result of injury during a game. Masterton fell backwards headfirst onto the ice after a body check. Masterton was not wearing a helmet and he suffered a massive brain hemorrhage. No operation was performed. Masteron died 27 hours after the injury. Of note, Masterton did not wear a helmet, which was routine for his era ("Masterton Dies of Head Injuries").

In 1972, Paul Fendley, a member of the junior ice hockey team the Guelph CMCs, died at the age of 19, approximately 3 days after striking ice his head on the ice. Fendley was checked by an opponent while handling the puck during play. As he lost balance his helmet came free, exposing his head. He struck the back of his head on the ice. Of note, Fendley had lost consciousness due to a hit a few days earlier. Whether or not this was a case of Second Impact Syndrome is speculative (Saxon, 2007).

The first documented death due to an ice hockey fight occurred in 2009. Don Sanderson, a senior league ice hockey player, was killed during a regular season game at the age of 21. After severalpunches were exchanged between both players, Sanderson's helmet slipped off and he stumbled to the ice, subsequently hitting his head on the ice and fracturing his skull. Sanderson transiently lost consciousness. After a matter of hours, Sanderson was comatose. He underwent surgery and remained in a coma for 3 weeks until succumbing to his injuries. Sanderson presumably suffered an epidural hematoma, but no autopsy report was available from gathered articles (CBC Sports).

CONCLUSION

In our thorough review of the literature on CNS injuries in ice hockey players, the following injuries were the most common: concussion (0.2 to 6.6 per 1000 player hours) and spinal cord injury (5 per 1000 player hours). Other rare injuries of undetermined incidence include: second impact syndrome, subarachnoid hemorrhage, subdural hematoma, epidural hematoma, spinal cord concussion, and vertebral hemorrhage. Controversial associations with long term consequences of head impact in ice hockey include Post-Concussive Syndrome and Chronic Traumatic Encephalopathy (CTE).

This literature search can serve as a valuable tool for health care practitioners and others who care for ice hockey players. Of note, we found that body checks from behind resulting in head contact with the boards can result in severe concussion and spinal cord injury. While helmets are essential in protecting the brain and face, the neck remains exposed and vulnerable to rare cervical spinal cord and vascular injuries. The allowance of fighting in the sport of ice hockey remains controversial. While the majority of fights end without serious injury, there are cases of concussion and even death associated with fighting. Long term consequences of repetitive head trauma are concerning with the discovery of CTE in multiple professional ice hockey players. Further education regarding the risks of the sport are necessary to prevent further neurological injuries.

Conflicts of Interest

This research received no funding and has no conflicts of interest to declare.

References

Benson, B. W., et al. (2011) A Prospective Study of Concussions among National Hockey League Players during Regular Season Games: The NHL-NHLPA Concussion Program. *CMAJ: Canadian Medical Association journal = journal de l'Association medicale canadienne.* 183.8: 905-11.

Boden, B. P., and C. G. Jarvis. (2009) Spinal Injuries in Sports. *Physical Medicine and Rehabilitation Clinics of North America.* 20.1: 55,68, vii.

CBC Sports. (Jan 2 2009) . Senior hockey league player dies from fight-related injury [http://www.cbc.ca/sports/hockey/senior-hockey-league-player-dies-from-fight-related-injury-1.793185].

Donaldson, L., M. Asbridgc, and M. D. Cusimano. (2013). Bodychccking Rules and Concussion in Elite Hockey. *PloS one.* 8.7: e69122.

ESPN 2011. (Dec 6 2011). Researcher: Bob Probert had CTE. [http://sports.espn.go.com/nhl/news/story?id=6177474].

Gerberich, S. G., et al. (1987). An Epidemiological Study of High School Ice Hockey Injuries. *Child's nervous system: ChNS: official journal of the International Society for Pediatric Neurosurgery.* 3.2: 59-64.

Honey, C. R. (1998). Brain Injury in Ice Hockey. *Clinical journal of sport medicine: official journal of the Canadian Academy of Sport Medicine* 8.1: 43-6.

McCrory, P. R., and S. F. Berkovic. (1998). Second Impact Syndrome. *Neurology.* 50.3: 677-83.

McKee, A. C., et al. (2013). The Spectrum of Disease in Chronic Traumatic Encephalopathy. *Brain: a journal of neurology.* 136.Pt 1: 43-64.

Sahjpaul, R. L., et al. (1998).Fatal Traumatic Vertebral Artery Aneurysm Rupture. Case Report." *Journal of neurosurgery.* 89.5: 822-4.

Saxon, Tony. (2007). Spirit of 72. *Guelph Mercury Staff.* [http://melosprogbazaar.com /index.php?topic=11304.0] ed.December 8.

Tator, C. H., and V. E. Edmonds. (1984). National Survey of Spinal Injuries in Hockey Players. *Canadian Medical Association journal.* 130.7: 875-80.

Tator, C. H., et al. (2004). Spinal Injuries in Canadian Ice Hockey: Documentation of Injuries Sustained from 1943-1999. *The Canadian journal of neurological sciences. Le journal canadien des sciences neurologiques.* 31.4: 460-6.

Unknown Author. (1907). Hockey Player Succumbs. *Ottawa Sun.* [http://news.google.com/newspapers?nid=2194&dat=19070307&id=fFouAAAAIBAJ&sjid=3tgFAAAAIBAJ&pg=6615,4690880] ed.March 7.

Unknown Author. (1968). Masterton Dies of Head Injuries. *St. Paul Dispatch.* [[http://www.northstarshockey.com/clip1.htm] ed.January 15.

USA Hockey. (2014) Membership Statistics. [http://www.usahockey.com/page/show /839306-membership-statistics].

Winder, M. J., K. Brett, and R. J. Hurlbert. (2011) Spinal Cord Concussion in a Professional Ice Hockey Player. *Journal of neurosurgery.Spine.* 14.5: 677-80.

In: Sports Injuries
Editor: Gabrielle Hopkins

ISBN: 978-1-63463-305-5

Chapter 3

PROTECTIVE HEADGEAR FOR RUGBY, AUSTRALIAN RULES FOOTBALL AND SOCCER

Con Hrysomallis, Ph.D.•
Institute of Sport, Exercise and Active Living,
College of Sport and Exercise Science, Victoria University,
Melbourne, Australia

ABSTRACT

Rugby, Australian Rules football (ARF) and soccer have high participation rates in numerous countries. A consequence of contact and collision sports is a notable injury rate and of particular concern is head injury, especially concussion. A countermeasure intended to reduce head injury prevalence in these football codes is non-obligatory protective soft-shell headgear. The adoption rate of this type of headgear for rugby (7 to 27%) was found to be higher than for ARF (2 to 8%). The main reason given for not wearing headgear was discomfort. Laboratory studies of soccer headgear demonstrated significant impact attenuation during scenarios simulating head to head contact. Laboratory studies of ARF and rugby headgear have shown that thickness is directly related to impact attenuation and that the type of headform and impact surface greatly influences the test results. Randomised controlled trials with teenage

• E-mail: con.hrysomallis@vu.edu.au.

rugby union players did not find headgear significantly reduced concussion rate or other head injuries. There was one attempted randomised controlled trial with ARF but was unable to be completed because of poor compliance with wearing headgear; this is a major challenge for researchers. One retrospective study found that soccer headgear reduced the proportion of concussions for collegiate athletes. There is some evidence as well as inconsistent results from prospective and retrospective studies that headgear may reduce concussion or superficial head injuries in rugby. The weight of the evidence suggests that the headgear assessed so far cannot be relied on its own to significantly reduce concussion rate but should not be dismissed completely.

1. Introduction

Football codes such as rugby, Australian Rules football and soccer are highly popular in many countries throughout the world but as with other contact or collision sports, injuries do occur. Concerted effort is required to prevent and manage injuries, particularly head injuries like concussion. Concerns have been raised about the short-term and potential long-term consequences of repeated concussions and even sub-concussive impacts [1, 2]. One approach to try and reduce head injury incidence and severity in sport is the utilisation of protective equipment. Non-mandatory padded headgear as opposed to hard-shell helmets have been approved for these football codes by the sport governing bodies [3-5] as long as they don't pose an injury hazard to any player. While not main stream practise, there are reports of sporting clubs and schools requiring their junior athletes wear protective headgear while playing rugby, ARF or soccer [6-8]. There are also cases of professional athletes in these sports who wear headgear on return to play following face or skull fractures or concussion [9-12]. Sustaining repeated concussions has been reported as contributing to the retirement of athletes from professional soccer among other sports [13].

Sports medicine and public interest in protective headgear is usually intensified after media reports of high-profile or junior athletes sustaining head injury while participating in the football codes without compulsory headgear [14]. There is a need to synthesise the current body of knowledge related to protective headgear for these football codes so as to assist those involved to make informed decisions as to the role of non-obligatory protective equipment. The objectives of this review are to (1) describe the adoption rates and attitudes to non-mandatory protective headgear in rugby, ARF and soccer; (2) report on the biomechanical evaluation of the headgear; (3) evaluate the effectiveness of the headgear on injury incidence; and (4) identify areas for future research. The review was centred on peer-reviewed journal articles identified from electronic literature searches using MEDLINE, CINAHL and SPORTDiscus databases up to September 2013, using the following search terms in various groupings: 'headgear', 'head guard', 'head protector', 'helmet', 'rugby', 'Australian', 'football', 'soccer', 'head', ' injuries' and 'concussion'. Additional studies were identified from the cited reference lists of the articles found by the electronic searches.

2. Head Injury Incidence

Head injuries in sport may encompass an injury spectrum range from superficial soft tissue such as lacerations and abrasions, through to concussion, skull fractures and uncommon catastrophic brain injuries such as sub-dural haematoma and intracranial haemorrhage [15]. The incidence of head injury in rugby, ARF and soccer has recently been reviewed and reported. Head injuries in soccer across all levels of play accounted for 4 to 20% of all injuries while concussion accounted for 3%, with a rate of 0.06/1000 hr for professional European soccer, 0.59 per 1000 hr for high school level and 1.08 per 1000 hr at the college level [16]. For ARF, at the community level the incidence of head injuries was 2.6/1000 hr, with concussion accounting for 4.3% of all injuries; at the elite level, concussion was one of the most common injuries with an incidence rate of 5 to 6/1000 hr [17] and multiple concussions to the same player throughout their career was not infrequent [18]. Rugby also had a notable proportion of head injuries, 14 to 25%, with concussion accounting for 5 to 15% of all injuries and occurring at a rate of 6.9/1000 hr for adolescents [16].

3. Protective Headgear

Headgear are designed to attenuate impact energy and distribute impact force applied to the head, usually achieved by energy-absorbing material such as a closed-cell foam liner compressing to absorb force, decreasing force to the head which reduces acceleration of the head. If the headgear can reduce head impact force and acceleration to below injury tolerance levels under sport specific impact scenarios then they can reduce injury risk [15]. There are a number of considerations that go into the design and construction of protective headgear and often there is a trade-off in certain parameters because of conflicting requirements. For instance, the need for a fastening system at the back, ventilation, uninterrupted vision and cut out sections over the ears for hearing will compromise coverage to certain parts of the head for rugby and ARF headgear. Other requisites usually include: the need to be flexible to conform to the contours of the head for a stable and comfortable fit; lightweight; aesthetics; affordability; and resilience to be able to withstand multiple impacts.

Recently, protective headgear has been designed for use in soccer, particularly for young male and female players [7]. Most of the soccer headgear resembles an enlarged headband, so their low profile is unlike the traditional 'helmet' look. There is usually an impact absorbing foam encased in an exterior fabric and sometimes with plastic inserts. Design considerations include protection of the impact areas such as the forehead and temple, lightweight, ventilation, moisture absorbing, adjustable fit and possibly ports to accommodate ponytails and other hair wearing options. Although the majority of soccer headgear has a low profile design, they are the more traditional fuller coverage headgear, one version resembled that used in martial arts [19] and others are rugby-type headgear that have been worn by players that have suffered severe concussion [12] or skull fracture [9].

4. Utilisation and Attitudes to Non-Mandatory Headgear

There have been a number of studies on the use and attitudes to protective headgear in rugby and ARF (Table 1) with many investigating a range of playing levels [8, 20, 22, 25], age groups [8, 20, 22-25] or gender [8, 20, 22]. All but one of the studies [22] was of retrospective design and the examined period for the majority of the studies was the previous playing season [20, 21, 23, 24]. There were 5 studies surveying rugby participants [8, 20-22, 25] and 2 studies on ARF [23, 24]. No published studies on the usage rate and attitudes to soccer protective headgear were found, possibly because of the recency of their utilisation in the sport.

Table 1. Adoption rates and attitudes to voluntary usage of protective headgear

Study (year)	Sport, level, participants	Study design	Percentage that were headgear	Main reasons for wearing headgear	Main reasons for not wearing headgear
Gerrard et al. (1994) [20]	RU, club level senior A, B, men, senior women, U/21, school boys and girls. 250 M 92 F	Retrospective questionnaire at the end of 1992 season	20%	To prevent injury (57%); because of previous injury (53%); based on medical advice (21%). Could give more than 1 reason	Not reported
Finch et al. (2001) [21]	RU, 10 randomly selected school teams, U/15. 139 M	6 teams assigned headgear. Survey at the end of the 1999 season.	79% Data collected during a trial of headgear	Feel safer (54%) Did not want to get an injury (42%).	Discomfort (61%)
Marshall et al. (2001) [22]	RU, club level senior A, B, men, senior women, U/21, school boys and girls. 240 M, 87 F	Prospective, weekly interviews during 1993 season	14% overall. School boys 33%. Loose forwards position highest users 23.5%	To prevent injury and because of past injury.	Not reported
Pettersen (2002) [8]	RU, high school, university, community, national. 39 M, 24 F players and 7 M, 2 F coaches.	Questionnaire on headgear and effectiveness on preventing concussion	27% overall (most of these from the national team 10/17)	62% of players and 33% of coaches thought it could prevent concussion.	Not mandatory, uncomfortable and expensive
Study (year)	Sport, level, participants	Study design	Percentage that wore headgear	Main reasons for wearing headgear	Main reasons for not wearing headgear
Finch et al. (2003) [23]	ARF, community-level, 3 senior and 1 junior teams, 70 M	Pilot study, retrospective questionnaire at the end of the 2000 season	8%	To prevent injury. 80% of non-users would wear one if they had an injury and 36% if it prevented injuries	Discomfort (47%), didn't like wearing it (42%) and didn't need to (23%).

Table 1. (Continued)

Study (year)	Sport, level, participants	Study design	Percentage that wore headgear	Main reasons for wearing headgear	Main reasons for not wearing headgear
Braham et al. (2004) [24]	ARF, community-level, senior and junior, 301 M	Retrospective questionnaire at the end of the 2000 season	2%	Safety and protection of previous injury. 67% of non-user would wear one if they had an injury, 32% if it was mandatory by their club and 26% if it prevented injury.	Didn't like wearing it (45%) and discomfort (41%)
Comstock et al. (2005) [25]	RU, tournament with varied levels of play, adults, 234 F	Retrospective questionnaire on most recent 3 months of play	7% (only forwards always worn headgear)	Injury prevention (85%)	Not reported

ARF = Australian Rules football; F=female; M=male; RU=rugby union; U = under.

The general overall adoption rate of protective headgear in rugby ranged from 7 to 27% [8, 20, 22, 25] and was higher than that for ARF 2 to 8% [23, 24]. There was one study [21] that reported a usage rate of 79% for school boys' rugby but this was for a trial that provided the headgear as part of the investigation so the figure is a vast overestimation of the general wearing rate.

One reason for the lesser rate of headgear usage in ARF could be the perceived risk of head injury by most ARF participants is lower and therefore there is no compelling motivation to wear headgear [23]. Playing position influenced headgear usage in rugby with forwards for both genders more likely to wear them because of their greater injury risk [22, 25]. Males were more likely to adopt headgear than female rugby participants probably due to their different styles of play, higher impact forces and injury incidence [22].

Not surprisingly, the main reason the participants gave for wearing headgear was to prevent injury [20-25]. Also featuring prominently as a reason for headgear usage was a previous injury [20, 22, 24]. This might allow participants to continue to play before full recovery from an injury, prevent the injury becoming more severe or avert recurrent injury [25]. The main reason given for not wearing headgear was discomfort [8, 21, 23, 24]. Other prominent reasons given were didn't need to or non-mandatory [8, 23]. Although discomfort was cited as a leading reason for not wearing headgear, improvement in comfort was not stated as a key factor that may sway non-users to adopt headgear. The primary incentives for a number of ARF participants that did not wear headgear to wear one would be if they had an injury or if it prevented injuries [23, 24].

5. Biomechanical Assessment of Impact Attenuation of Soccer Protective Headgear

Soccer is unique in the regard that it is the only contact sport that purposefully uses the head to control and progress the ball [26]. Early concerns in soccer were that repetitive heading, particularly by younger players, may be a risk factor for cognitive impairment, so the initial focus was to evaluate the soccer protective headgear in experimental set ups that simulated the conditions of soccer heading [7, 27]. It can be seen from Table 2 that there have been four laboratory studies on impact attenuation of soccer headgear during heading a soccer ball [7, 19, 27, 28]. Tests have been reported on six brands of headgear: Soccer Docs; Kangaroo which was similar to martial arts headgear, foam liner encased in vinyl, overall thickness about 20mm, forehead region 28 mm [19]; Head Blast had foam with thin plastic sheet embedded, fabric backing, plastic front cover, about 8 mm thick [19]; Head'r; Full90 (Headers) comprised of foam bound to fabric exterior, about 11 mm thick [19]; and Protector which had a hard plastic insert backed with foam within terry-cloth headband and similar thickness to Headers [7]. Details of the type of foam and densities in the headgear were not available.

The testing methods have involved the use of surrogate headforms [19, 27] or a force platform [7] with ball contact speeds ranging from 9 to 30 $m.s^{-1}$ and human volunteers tests with low speed ball contacts of 6 to 9. 8 $m.s^{-1}$ [19, 28]. The lower ball speeds have been reported as being common in general soccer play and heading [7, 27]. Three of the studies [7, 27, 28] found that headgear could reduce peak acceleration or force by 11 to 17% but they only considered linear acceleration from ball contact and the findings may be gender specific. Female volunteers actually experiencing greater head acceleration while wearing headgear possibly because of their less head mass and neck strength which may partially explain the greater incidence of concussion in female soccer players than male [28]. The one study [19] that reported no significant reduction in impacts from ball contact used the most biofidelic headform, highest ball speeds, considered rotational acceleration in its injury index and surmised that headgear was ineffective for head to ball contact because of the large amount of ball deformation relative to headgear thickness. Two of the studies [19, 27] which included tests on the Kangaroo brand headgear that was twice as thick as all the others, blinded their results so comparison between brands was limited. One study [7] found that all 3 brands tested Headers, Head Blast and Protector reduced impact with no difference between them. Another study [28] found that during tests with male volunteers the slightly thicker Full90 headgear displayed a greater reduction in linear acceleration than the Head Blast headgear. It is important to note that overall, the accelerations, injuries indices and risk of head injury from the ball contact testing with and without headgear were low [19, 28]. Heading the ball may be considered low acute injury risk compared to head contact with rigid body parts. One study [19] simulated head to head clashes which along with contact with other body parts or the ground is now realised to be a more likely

Table 2. Laboratory evaluation of impact attenuation of soccer protective headgear

Study (year)	Headgear brand	Laboratory test	Significant findings ($p<0.05$)
Naunheim at el. (2003) [27]	Soccer Docs, Kangaroo, Head Blast, Head'r	Headgear placed on rigid magnesium headform with triaxial accelerometer and flexible neck; high and low pressure soccer balls projected at 9, 12, and 15 $m.s^{-1}$. Five trials for each headgear and bare headform (control)	Peak acceleration values with and without headgear were very low (15 to 30 g). Headgear reduced peak acceleration (12 to 17%) at highest speed and pressure. No difference or protection at low or moderate speeds or low pressure.
Broglio et al. (2003) [7]	Headers (name now changed to Full90), Head Blast, Protector	Headgear attached to a vertically mounted forceplate and soccer balls projected at 15.6 $m.s^{-1}$. Fifty trials on each headgear and bare forceplate (control)	All 3 reduced peak force (11 to 13%) with no difference between them. Protector reduced time to peak force (23%) and impulse (11%). Full90 increased impulse (5%).
Withnall et al. (2005) [19]	Full90, Head Blast, Kangaroo	Headgear attached to Hybrid III headform and neck which measured linear and angular acceleration while impacting another Hybrid III headform at two sites at 2 to 5 $m.s^{-1}$; ball impacts with headgear at 10,20 and 30 $m.s^{-1}$; human volunteer with a bite plate with accelerometers heading a ball at low speeds of 6 and 8 $m.s^{-1}$	Headgear on average reduced head to head impact peak acceleration and HIPmax by 33%; maximum bare head acceleration was 169 g. Accelerations (15 to 60 g), HIPmax and concussion risk from ball impacts with and without head gear were generally very low. No overall significant reduction in impacts from ball contact for Hybrid III or volunteer tests.
Tierney et al. (2008) [28]	Head Blast, Full90	Headgear was worn by 44 volunteers (29 women, 15 men) with a mouthpiece triaxial accelerometer while heading a ball projected at 9.8 $m.s^{-1}$ Heading was also done without headgear (control)	Overall, peak acceleration (15 to 22 g) and HIC (14 to 20) values with and without headgear were very low. Head Blast reduced linear acceleration by 11% and Full 90 by 17% for men. Headgear increased acceleration by 7 to 8% for women. Women showed greater head acceleration (10 to 44%) than men with headgear and without.

HIC = Head Injury Criteria; HIPmax= Head Impact Power.

mechanism for concussion than heading the soccer ball [29, 30]. It was demonstrated that headgear reduced acceleration and the index for mild brain injury by a third during head clashes and it was concluded that headgear was effective in reducing impact between two stiff objects such as in head to head contact [19].

There is a standard for testing headgear used in soccer [31]. Drop tests are conducted with a Hybrid III headform and neck assembly, total mass of 8.8 kg and the resultant linear acceleration is measured. The impact area is an angled 50 mm band encircling the head. Three different impact scenarios are considered, heading the ball impacts are not addressed. The first test is an impact at 2.0 $m.s^{-1}$ with a steel post anvil to represent a goal post. The second test involves impact at 3.8 $m.s^{-1}$ with another Hybrid III headform. The final scenario is impact at 2.5 $m.s^{-1}$ with a firm modular elastomer programmer (MEP) pad on top of an anvil to simulate contact with the ground.

For all 3 test scenarios, the peak linear acceleration should not exceed 80 g. The standard also specifies a multiple impact test on the MEP pad; 5 impacts on the same spot with 75 s intervals and the peak acceleration of the final drop should not exceed 15% of the first drop. The second test scenario of the standard was similar to that used by one of the laboratory studies [19] which found that at an impact speed of 4 $m.s^{-1}$ only one of the 3 headgear tested did not exceed a peak acceleration value of 80 g. This study included a headgear that was twice as thick as the other two but since the data was blinded, the characteristics of the best performing headgear could not be confirmed.

6. Biomechanical Assessment of Impact Attenuation of Rugby and ARF Protective Headgear

Several headgear for rugby and ARF have undergone biomechanical testing with the majority originally intended for rugby (Table 3). The two studies [32, 34] that evaluated the most headgear blinded the brand names but some information on construction and composition was available. The thickness of the headgear ranged from 7 [33] to 16 mm [35], ethyl vinyl acetate [34] or polyethylene [35] foam were commonly used and foam density ranged from 48 to 87 $kg.m^{-3}$ [34].

Table 3. Laboratory evaluation of impact attenuation of rugby and ARF protective headgear

Study (year)	Headgear	Laboratory test	Significant findings ($p<0.05$)
McIntosh and McCrory (2000) [32]	8 headgear from 6 manufacturers. Brand names blinded, limited details on composition.	Headgear attached to both rigid magnesium and Hybrid III headforms and impacted a rigid anvil at speeds of 2 to 3.4 $m.s^{-1}$; impact energies of 9.8 to 29.4 J. 5 repeated drops at same site with impact speed of 2.4 $m.s^{-1}$ also conducted.	For impact speeds of 3.1 $m.s^{-1}$ and greater, all headgear exceeded the proposed acceleration (150 g) and HIC (1000) thresholds and deemed unlikely to prevent concussion. Repeated drops increased peak acceleration from 5 to 50%.
Knouse et al. (2003) [33]	2 types of rugby headgear, 10 samples of each: Canterbury Honeycomb 10 mm thick, high-density closed-cell foam and 96 grams; Gilbert Vanguard 7 to 8 mm thick, larger continuous sections and 74 grams	Headgear attached to Hybrid III headform and impacted a MEP pad on top of an anvil at a speed of 2.4 $m.s^{-1}$ 10 repeated drops on the side and back of the headgear also conducted.	Highest peak acceleration (116 g) and GSI (419) values were all lower than those assumed to cause head injury. Side of the headgear offered greater impact attenuation than the back. Repetitive drops increased peak acceleration from 11 to 56%
Hrysomallis (2004) [34]	7 rugby and ARF headgear, brand names blinded: thickness ranged from 8 to 15 mm, all comprised of ethyl vinyl acetate foam with a general density range of 48 to 87 $kg.m^{-3}$	Headgear attached to NOCSAE headform and impacted a 1.3 cm MEP pad on top of an anvil at a speed of 4.1 $m.s^{-1}$; impact energy of 56 J. Impacts to the front, side and top were conducted.	Headgear on average reduced HIC values by about 50% compare to bare headform impacts. Headgear thickness correlated with HIC values for side impacts ($r=-0.8$). Best performing headgear had the greatest thickness and foam density and only one to register HIC values of less than 1000 and peak accelerations less than 200 g for side and front impacts.
McIntosh et al.(2004) [35]	Albion Headpro model for ARF, modified: 12.5 mm thick polyethylene foam density of 65 $kg.m^{-3}$ plus 2 mm ethylene vinyl acetate insert; Canterbury Honeycomb for rugby, standard: 10 mm thick 45 $kg.m^{-3}$ polyethylene foam; Canterbury Honeycomb, modified: 16 mm thick 60 $kg.m^{-3}$ polyethylene foam	Headgear attached to a rigid magnesium headform and impacted a rigid anvil on the front and side at speeds of 2.4 to 3.4 $m.s^{-1}$; impact energies of 14.7 to 29.4 J. Six repeated impacts to same site also conducted.	The modified, thicker Canterbury headgear reduced peak acceleration by about 75% to 78% for side impacts to below 200 g at 2.4 and 2.8 $m.s^{-1}$. Albion outperformed the Honeycomb at 3.1 and 3.4 $m.s^{-1}$ but both tended to exceed 200 g. Repeated impacts at the same lateral site at 3.4 $m.s^{-1}$ increased peak acceleration by 21 to 51%.

g = acceleration of 9.8 $m.s^{-2}$; GSI = Gadd Severity Index; HIC = Head Injury Criteria; J = Joules; MEP = Modular Elastomer Programmer; NOCSAE = National Operating Committee on Standards for Athletic Equipment.

The headforms used to measure linear acceleration for the impact tests have been rigid magnesium [32, 35], Hybrid III [32, 33] or NOCSAE [34], with the latter two yielding headforms considered to be more biofidelic [36]. The impacting surface has been either a rigid steel anvil [32, 35] or a firm 1.3 cm MEP pad on top of the anvil intended to simulate the playing surface [31]. Since the side of the head has been identified as the most frequent location for impacts that produce concussion in rugby and ARF [37], this site is a commonly assessed region of headgear; tests have also been carried out to the front and top of the headgear. Impacts have been performed to the back of the headgear [33] but because of the posterior fastening design of most headgear, this comprises the amount of padding [34] and protection at this region [33]. Impact speeds during drop tests ranged from 2 to 4.1 $m.s^{-1}$ [32, 34] with 2.4 $m.s^{-1}$ being frequently included [32, 33, 35] because the testing was aligned with the International Rugby Board (IRB) standard for headgear [5] that specified a drop height of 30 cm which produced that impact speed. It is now acknowledged that the impact speeds in sport may be greater than those simulated in these tests [35]. The highest test speed utilised 4.1 $m.s^{-1}$ was to generate an impact energy of 56 J [34] that had been shown to result in concussion in ARF or rugby [37]. Peak linear acceleration of the headform has been the primary parameter investigated; other parameters which have been used as injury risk indicators such as GSI [33] and HIC [32, 34] are derived from the impact acceleration and include a temporal component. One of the limitations of the testing was it did not account for rotational acceleration which along with translational acceleration [38] can produce head injuries such as concussion [39]. Doubt has been raised as to whether protective headgear can decrease rotation [16] but limited investigation has been conducted in this area. There is some indirect support that headgear can influence rotation from the only laboratory assessment [19] that consider rotational acceleration in its head injury index and found that soccer protective headgear reduced it by 33%.

Protective headgear can reduce the magnitude of the impact acceleration and related injury indices but whether the reduction is sufficient to significantly reduce injury risk is open to interpretation. The first investigation [32] into the performance of rugby and ARF headgear concluded that they were unlikely to lessen the probability of head injury such as concussion. The type of headform and impact surface has a dramatic effect on the test results and whether the headgear is deemed likely to prevent injury. This can be illustrated by comparing the acceleration values generated when the same headgear is tested using rigid and non-rigid components. The standard

Canterbury Honeycomb headgear was assessed in one study [35] using a rigid magnesium headform impacting a steel anvil at 2.4 $m.s^{-1}$ and for a side impact produced peak acceleration of 276 g and for 6 repeated impacts on the same site generated peak acceleration of 399 g. If 200 g was considered the injury threshold then this headgear would be considered inadequate to reduce injury risk. When the same headgear was evaluated in another study [33] using the Hybrid III headform impacting a 1.3 cm MEP pad on top of the steel anvil at the same speed and site, the peak acceleration was 44 g and after 10 repeated impacts it was 70 g, well below 200g and only 16 to 17.5% of the acceleration values from tests with the rigid components.

Headgear thickness was related to impact attenuation capability. The best performing headgear had the thickest padding and high density foam [34, 35] and it appears that headgear needs to be at least 15 mm thick to have any scope of providing adequate protection. The design and construction can influence fit and impact dissipation; the honeycomb configuration with small, individual geometrical sections of padding may be more flexible and allow for a better fit while headgear with longer, continuous sections of padding may be better at dissipating impact over a greater area [35]. The impact energy attenuating foam used in the headgear needs to be resilient because of the prospect of receiving repetitive impacts. Test results revealed that repeated impacts to the same site may increase acceleration by up to 50% or more [32, 33, 35], indicating that the foam does not reconfigure to its original thickness but remains slightly compressed, decreasing its impact attenuating capacity. Most of the headgear assessed to date has comprised of closed-cell foams. Future research should consider evaluating other materials, for instance, Sorbothane®, a viscoelastic polyether-based polyurethane which has recently been incorporated into headgear [40].

The only standard that is related to headgear used in rugby or ARF is by the IRB which is the world governing and law-making body of the game of rugby union [5]. The regulations for IRB approved headgear stipulate that the headgear cannot be thicker than 10 mm or have a foam density greater than 45 $kg.m^{-3}$. When the headgear is attached to a rigid headform and dropped from a height of 30 mm onto a rigid anvil at an impact speed of 2.4 $m.s^{-1}$, the resultant peak acceleration should not be less than 200 kg. The standard actually limits the impact attenuation ability of the headgear for rugby union. Headgear approved by this standard are intended to be effective against superficial head injuries but have insufficient padding and offer minimal protection against more severe head injuries such as concussion. The intention is likely to be that rugby union players don't feel invincible with the IRB approved headgear and engage in risky behaviour. It has been recognised that the absence of a well-conceived international standard for headgear for rugby and ARF creates a deficiency in the pursuit to appraise headgear and avert the gamut of head injuries, particularly concussion [32]. Due to the complex nature, there remains deliberation about injury tolerance levels but it has recently been proposed that for headgear to be effective in reducing concussion risk in Australian football they would need to protect against head change in velocities of up to 7 $m.s^{-1}$ and reduce head resultant linear and angular acceleration to below 50 g and 1500 $rad.s^{-2}$, respectively [41]. Further research is required to fully establish validated injury tolerance levels for concussion in the various football codes, which would include the incorporation of rotational acceleration.

7. Influence of Protective Headgear on Head Injury Rate

There have been a number of studies on the effect of headgear on head injury occurrence with the vast majority involving rugby union (Table 4). There has been only one investigation on soccer [48], one attempted on ARF [44] and none reported for rugby league. For soccer there is low-level evidence from a retrospective, cross-sectional study of adolescent soccer players that found soccer headgear use was associated with about a 60% reduction in the risk of sustaining a concussion and reduced risk of other head injuries [48]. The findings needs to be considered in light of the limitations of the study design, it involved only one soccer club, headgear use was not randomised and there was a reliance on memory recall to report injuries.

The intended controlled trial on the effectiveness of headgear for ARF [44] was unable to be completed because of the low adoption rate of headgear by the participants. This highlights that compliance is a major challenge for researchers when attempting to investigate the efficacy of non-mandatory protective equipment. In spite of this potential obstacle, prospective, controlled trials have been conducted with teenage rugby union participants [42, 49]. The first study [42] provided headgear to the intervention group if they weren't already wearing their own. It was found that the players that wore headgear did not show a significant reduction in concussion rate but it was

Table 4. Epidemiological studies of the influence of protective headgear on head injury rate

Study (year)	Sport, level, participants	Study design	Headgear details	Head injuries	Significant findings ($p<0.05$)
McIntosh and McCrory (2001) [42]	Rugby union, U/15 A grade, 16 teams, 294 M	Prospective , controlled, 1 season, 1179 player exposures with headgear and 357 without	Albion Body Pro or Madison Elite Rugby or their own	Concussion	Headgear did not reduce concussion rate
Jones et al. (2004) [43]	Rugby union, i) Emergency department presentations, 164 cases. ii) 1999 Rugby World Cup, 20 national teams, 547 M	i) Case-control study: cases being injured players (12.3 % headgear wearers) and controls (21 % headgear wearers) being same position opponent ii) Cohort study: video review, 41 games, 277 player exposures with headgear and 1333 without	Not reported	Head and face lacerations, abrasions or fractures	i) Headgear did not reduce injuries ii) Headgear decreased risk of bleeding head injuries among forwards (OR = 0.14, 95% CI 0.01 to 0.99)
Braham and Finch (2004) [44]	ARF, community-level, 23 senior and junior teams, 301 M	Clustered RCT, 1 season, 4 groups: headgear, mouthguard, headgear and mouth guard and control	Not reported		Unable to access effectiveness due to very low compliance with wearing headgear
Marshall et al. (2005) [45]	Rugby union, club level senior A, B, men, senior women, U/21, school boys. 240 M, 87 F	Prospective, cross-sectional, 1 season	Not reported	Orofacial, scalp, ears, concussion	Headgear reduced risk of scalp and ear injuries (RR = 0.59, 95% CI 0.19 to 1.86) Headgear did not reduce concussion risk
Kahanov et al. (2005) [46]	Rugby union, collegiate level from 8 universities, 131 M	Retrospective, cross-sectional, 49% headgear wearers, 51% non-wearers	Not reported	Concussion	Decreased portion of concussions for headgear wearers (24%) versus non-wearers (76%) and reduced severity

Table 4. (Continued)

Study (year)	Sport, level, participants	Study design	Headgear details	Head injuries	Significant findings ($p<0.05$)
Kemp et al. (2008) [47]	Rugby union, 13 professional clubs, 757 M	Prospective, cross-sectional, 3 seasons	Not reported	Concussion, head and facial fractures and lacerations	Headgear reduced incidence of concussion (2.0/1000 player-hr versus 4.6) and head injury in general
Delaney et al. (2008) [48]	Soccer, 12 to 17 yr olds, 1 club, 180 M, 98 F	Retrospective, cross-sectional, 1 season, 52 headgear wearers, 216 non-wearers	Headband configuration, no chin strap	Concussion, Head abrasions, laceration or contusions	Headgear reduced risk of concussion (RR = 0.38) and other head injuries
McIntosh et al. (2009) [49]	Rugby union, U13 to U20 M, 82 teams in season 1, 87 teams in season 2	Cluster RCT, 2 seasons, 1493 control, 1128 standard headgear wearers, 1474 modified headgear wearers	Standard headgear = 10 mm thick, 45 $kg.m^{-3}$ foam; modified headgear = 16 mm thick, 60 $kg.m^{-3}$ foam	Concussion and head injury	Headgear did not reduce the risk or severity of concussion or head injury
Hollis et al. (2009) [50]	Rugby union, nonprofessional, 26 clubs, 8 schools, 15 years and older, 3207 M	Prospective, cross-sectional, 1 to 3 seasons, 36% headgear wearers	Not reported	Concussion	Headgear reduced the risk of concussion (RR = 0.57, 95% CI 0.40-0.82)
Chalmers et al. (2012) [51]	Rugby union, amateur, 13 years and older, 704 M	Prospective, cross-sectional, 1 season, 1807 player exposures with headgear and 4223 without	Not reported	Any injury during the game	Headgear associated with increased risk of game injury (RR = 1.23, 95% CI 1.00-1.50)

CI = confidence interval; F = female; M = male; OR = odds ratio; RCT = randomised controlled trial; U = under; RR = rate ratio.

acknowledged that for this study a small number of concussions were registered, 7 players wearing headgear sustained concussion and 2 players without.

The other study [49] was a clustered by teams RCT that had two intervention arms, one group was provided with standard headgear and the other group was provided with modified headgear that was thicker and denser. This high-level study design did not find that headgear reduced the rate or severity of concussion. Low compliance was recognised as limitation with only 11% of total player-game exposures with the modified headgear but there was 46% exposure with the standard headgear; informal feedback from the players was that the modified headgear was too stiff and hence uncomfortable. There is no high-level evidence from prospective controlled trials that protective headgear can reduce the incidence of concussion but there is some evidence from cross-sectional studies that headgear can influence concussion risk and other head injury risks.

In these cross-sectional studies, headgear use was not randomised, the players self-selected whether to wear headgear and details of the headgear were not recorded. It was shown in some studies that headgear reduced the rate of superficial head injuries such lacerations and abrasions for a range of playing levels from school boy to professional [43, 45, 47] but this finding was not universal [43, 49]. There has been one retrospective, cross-sectional investigation with collegiate players [46] that reported a 70% reduction in concussion associated with headgear use. Of the three prospective cross-sectional studies that monitored concussion rate, two studies [47, 50] found that headgear decreased the incidence of concussion from 43 to 57% and the other study [45] did not detect a protective effect. Overall, it would appear that the effect of protective headgear on the incidence on concussion in rugby is inconclusive. As for the influence of headgear on concussion severity, two prospective studies did not find a difference in the average severity for wearers and non-wearers [47, 49] while the one retrospective study reported a reduction in the severity of symptoms from 4 days to 2 days [46]. The weight of the evidence at the moment suggests that headgear may not influence the severity of concussion.

One of the investigations [51] reported the effect of headgear on any game injury and found that headgear was associated with a 23% greater risk of injury. Since the categorisation of injuries to specific body parts was not provided, it is unknown what effect headgear had on head injury rate but this study does highlight an important issue, 'risk compensation' [52]. That is, athletes may develop a false sense of security when wearing headgear, reduce inhibition and engage in more physically aggressive play that may actual increase the risk of injury [30]. Further investigation is required on this issue [49] but none of the epidemiological studies to date on rugby, soccer or ARF have reported a significantly higher incidence of head injuries for athletes wearing headgear.

CONCLUSION

Head injuries and in particular concussion are a concern for participants in rugby, ARF and soccer. Non-mandatory soft-shell protective headgear are available and have been approved for use by the sport governing bodies as long as they do not pose an injury risk to any player. The general utilisation rate of headgear was 7 to 27 % in rugby and 2 to 8% in ARF; figures for soccer were not available possibly because of the recency of their adoption in the sport. The main reason for not wearing protective headgear was discomfort. Biomechanical evaluation of soccer headgear general found that impact during heading a soccer ball could be attenuated but this situation was not the main mechanism for head injury in that sport. Head contact with a firm object was more likely to produce injury and test scenarios simulating head to head contact found that soccer headgear could significantly attenuate impact. Laboratory assessment of ARF and rugby headgear generally found that the greater the headgear thickness, the greater the impact attenuation. The test results were very much dependant on whether a rigid or yielding headform and impact surface were used. Further research is required to fully establish a laboratory test protocol with biofidelic components, injury tolerance levels and impact characteristics that are representative of those that result in injury in the sport. Epidemiological data from high-level study designs revealed headgear did not decrease concussion or other head injury rate in teenage rugby players. No data were available for the effectiveness of headgear on head injury rate in ARF. There was low-to-moderate level evidence from prospective and retrospective cross-sectional studies that headgear could reduce concussion or other head injuries in soccer and rugby but some inconsistent results were also reported.

The weight of the evidence suggests that the non-mandatory headgear assessed so far cannot be relied on its own to significantly reduce head injury rates but should not be dismissed completely. Whether advancements in technology and materials significantly enhance the impact attenuation of protective headgear will need to await future research. It follows that the most effective way to reduce head injuries is to limit the possibility of head contact in the first instance. At the moment, headgear may be more effective as part of a multifactorial approach to injury reduction which would include education on safe sporting practises, skills training, strict adherence to rules, enforcement of penalties for dangerous play and thorough management of previous head injuries.

REFERENCES

[1] Bailes J. E., Petraglia A. L., Omalu B. I., et al. Role of subconcussion in repetitive mild traumatic brain injury. *J. Neurosurg.*, 2013;119(5):1235-45.

[2] Nowinski C. Hit parade: the future of the sports concussion crisis. *Cerebrum*, 2013;2:1-11.

[3] Australian Football League. Laws of Australian Football 2013. 9.2 Prohibition of Items. http://www.afl.com.au/staticfile/AFL%20Tenant/AFL/Static%20Files/Laws-of-Australian-Football-2013.pdf. Accessed 9 Dec 2013.

[4] Fédération Internationale de Football Association. Laws of the Game. Law 4 – The players' equipment. http://www.fifa.com/mm/document/footballdevelopment/refereeing/81/42/36/log2013en_neutral.pdf. Accessed 9 Dec 2013.

[5] International Rugby Board. Regulation 12. Standard performance specifications for specific items of players' clothing. http://www.irb.com/lawregulations/regulations/ index.html. Accessed 8 Dec 2013.

[6] To helmet or not? Junior footy is divided on a vexed question. The Age, June 2 2012. http://www.theage.com.au/victoria/to-helmet-or-not-junior-footy-is-divided-on-a-vexed-question-20120601-1zng3.html. Accessed Dec 9 2013.

[7] Broglio S. P., Ju Y.-Y., Broglio M. D., et al. The efficacy of soccer headgear. *J. Athl. Train.*, 2003;38(3):220-4.

[8] Pettersen J. A. Does rugby headgear prevent concussion? Attitudes of Canadian players and coaches. *Br. J. Sports Med.*, 2002;36(1):19-22.

[9] Chelsea goalkeeper Petr Cech says headgear saved him from serious head injury against Fulham. The Telegraph, 27 Sept 2011. http://www.telegraph.co.uk/sport/football/teams/chelsea/8791195/Chelsea-goalkeeper-Petr-Cech-says-headgear-saved-him-from-serious-head-injury-against-Fulham.html. Accessed Dec 9 2013.

[10] Christian Chivu loves his helmet. Soccer Safari, March 16 2011. http://blog.ctnews.com/levitt/2011/03/16/christian-chivu-loves-his-helmet/. Accessed Dec. 9 2013.

[11] Carlton captain Marc Murphy targets Collingwood to return from broken cheekbone. Herald Sun, June 28 2013. http://www.heraldsun.com.au/sport/afl/carlton-captain-marc-murphy-targets-collingwood-to-return-from-broken-cheekbone/story-fni5f5nx-1226671622615. Accessed Dec 9 2013.

[12] Houston's Carr on long road to recovery from concussion. MLSsoccer.com, July 26 2011. http://www.mlssoccer.com/news/article/2011/07/26/houstons-carr-long-road-recovery-concussion. Accessed 9 Dec 2013.

[13] Jimmy Conrad Retires from MLS. The Goat Parade Aug. 17 2011. http://www.thegoatparade.com/2011/8/17/2369285/jimmy-conrad-retires-from-mls. Accessed Dec 9 2013.

[14] Hrysomallis C. Should helmets be used in AFL? The Conversation April 4 2011 [online]. http://theconversation.edu.au/shouldhelmets-be-used-in-afl-620. Accessed 9 Dec 2013.

[15] McIntosh A. S., McCrory P. Preventing head and neck injury. *Br. J. Sports Med.,* 2005;39(6):314-8.

[16] McIntosh A. S., Andersen T. E., Bahr R., et al. Sports helmets now and in the future. *Br. J. Sports Med.,* 2011;45(16):1258-65.

[17] Hrysomallis C. Injury incidence, risk factors and prevention in Australian Rules football. *Sports Med.,* 2013;43(5):339–54.

[18] King T., Rosenberg M., Braham R., et al. Life after the game – injury profile of past elite Australian football players. *J. Sci. Med. Sport*, 2013;16(4):302-6.

[19] Withnall C., Shewchenko N., Wonnacott M, et al. Effectiveness of headgear in football. *Br. J. Sports Med.*, 2005;39(Suppl. 1):i40-8.

[20] Gerrard D. F., Waller A. E., Bird Y. N. The New Zealand rugby injury and performance project: II. Previous injury experience of a rugby-playing cohort. *Br. J. Sports Med.,* 1994;28(4):229-33.

[21] Finch C. F., McIntosh A. S., McCrory P. What do under 15 year old schoolboy rugby union players think about protective headgear? *Br. J. Sports Med.*, 2001;35(2):89-94.

[22] Marshall S. W., Waller A. E., Loomis D. P., et al. Use of protective equipment in a cohort of rugby players. *Med. Sci. Sports Exerc.*, 2001;33(12):2131-8.

[23] Finch C. F., McIntosh A. S., McCrory P., et al. A pilot study of the attitudes of Australian Rules footballers towards protective headgear. *J. Sci. Med. Sport,* 2003;6(4): 505-11.

[24] Braham R. A., Finch C. F., McIntosh A., et al. Community football players' attitudes towards protective equipment – a pre-season measure. *Br. J. Sports Med.,* 2004;38(4): 426-30.

[25] Comstock R. D., Fields S. K., Knox C. L. Protective equipment use among female rugby players. *Clin. J. Sport Med.,* 2005;15(4):241-5.

[26] Kirkendall D. T., Jordan S. E., Garrett W. Heading and head injuries in soccer. *Sports Med.*, 2001;31(5):369-86.

[27] Naunheim R. S., Ryden A., Standeven J., et al. Does soccer headgear attenuate the impact when heading a soccer ball? *Acad. Emerg. Med.*, 2003;10(1):85-90.

[28] Tierney R. T., Higgins M., Caswell S. V., et al. Sex differences in head acceleration during heading while wearing soccer headgear. *J. Athl. Train.,* 2008;43(6):578-84.

[29] Gessel L. M., Fields S. K., Collins C. L., et al. Concussion among United States high school and collegiate athletes. *J. Athl. Train.,* 2007;42(4):495-503.

[30] Niedfeldt M. W. Head injuries, heading, and the use of headgear in soccer. *Curr. Sports Med. Rep.,* 2011;10(6):324-9.

[31] ASTM International. ASTM F2439-06 (2011) Standard specification for headgear used in soccer.

[32] McIntosh A. S., McCrory P. Impact energy attenuation performance of football headgear. *Br. J. Sports Med.,* 2000;34(5):337-41.

[33] Knouse C. L., Gould T. E., Caswell S. V., et al. Efficacy of rugby headgear in attenuating repetitive linear impact forces. *J. Athl. Train.*, 2003;38(4):330-5.

[34] Hrysomallis C. Impact energy attentuation of protective football headgear against a yielding surface. *J. Sci. Med. Sport,* 2004;7(2):156-64.

[35] McIntosh A., McCrory P., Finch C. F. Performance enhanced headgear: a scientific approach to the development of protective headgear. *Br. J. Sports Med.*, 2004;38(1):46-9.

[36] Hodgson V. R. National Operating Committee on Standards for Athletic Equipment football helmet certification program. *Med. Sci. Sports*, 1975;7(3):225-32.

[37] McIntosh A. S., McCrory P., Comerford J. The dynamics of concussive head impacts in rugby and Australian rules football. *Med. Sci. Sports Exerc.*, 2000;32(12):1980-4.

[38] Pellman E. J., Viano D. C., Tucker A. M., et al. Concussion in professional football: reconstruction of game impacts and injuries. *Neurosurg.,* 2003;53(4):799-814.

[39] Ommaya A. K., Gennarelli T. A. Cerebral concussion and traumatic unconsciousness. Correlation of experimental and clinical observations of blunt head injuries. *Brain,* 1974;97(4):633-54.

[40] Genesis headgear. http://madisonsport.com.au/rugby-protective/rugby-head-guards/ genesis-headguard. Accessed 12 Dec 2013.

[41] Benson B. W., McIntosh A. S., Maddocks D., et al. What are the most effective risk-reduction strategies in sport concussions? *Br. J. Sports Med.,* 2013;47(5):321-6.

[42] McIntosh A. S., McCrory P. Effectiveness of headgear in a pilot study of under 15 rugby union football. *Br. J. Sports Med.*, 2001;35(3):167-9.

[43] Jones S. J., Lyons R. A., Evans R., et al. Effectiveness of rugby headgear in preventing soft tissue injuries to the head: a case-control and video cohort study. *Br. J. Sports Med.*, 2004;38(2):159-62.

[44] Braham R. A., Finch C. F. Do community football players wear allocated protective equipment? Descriptive results from a randomised controlled trial. *J. Sci. Med. Sport,* 2004;7(2):216-20.

[45] Marshall S. W., Loomis D. P., Waller A. E., et al. Evaluation of protective equipment for prevention of injuries in rugby union. *Int. J. Epidemiol.*, 2005;34(1):113-8.

[46] Kahanov L., Dusa M. J., Wilkinson S., et al. Self-reported headgear use and concussions among collegiate men's rugby union players. *Res. Sports Med.,* 2005; 13(2): 77-89.

[47] Kemp S. P. T., Hudson Z., Brooks J. H. M., et al. The epidemiology of head injuries in English professional rugby union. *Clin. J. Sport Med.,* 2008;18(3):227-34.

[48] Delaney J. S., Al-Kashmiri A., Drummond R., et al. The effect of protective headgear on head injuries and concussions in adolescent football (soccer) players. *Br. J. Sports Med.,* 2008;42(2):110-5.

[49] McIntosh A., McCrory P., Finch C. F., et al. Does padded headgear prevent head injury in rugby union football? *Med. Sci. Sport Exerc.*, 2009;41(2):306-13.

[50] Hollis S. J., Stevenson M. R., McIntosh A. S., et al. Incidence, risk, and protective factors of mild traumatic brain injury in a cohort of Australian

nonprofessional male rugby players. *Am. J. Sports Med.,* 2009;37(12):2328-33.

[51] Chalmers D. J., Samaranayaka A., Gulliver P., et al. Risk factors for injury in rugby union football in New Zealand: a cohort study. *Br. J. Sports Med.,* 2012; 46(2): 95-102.

[52] Hagel B., Meeuwisse, W. Risk compensation: a "side effect" of sport injury prevention? *Clin. J. Sport Med.,* 2004;14(4):193-6.

In: Sports Injuries
Editor: Gabrielle Hopkins
ISBN: 978-1-63463-305-5

Chapter 4

PREDICTING AND PREVENTING SPORT INJURIES: THE ROLE OF STRESS

***Aurelio Olmedilla*[1,*]*, Víctor J. Rubio*[2] *and Enrique Ortega*[1]**
[1]University of Murcia, Murcia, Spain
[2]University Autonoma Madrid, Madrid, Spain

ABSTRACT

Hardly any sport practitioner would have finished his/her career without suffering at least one sport injury. Sport injury is a broadly spread out morbidity condition sustained as a result of an energy transfer when the specific tissue or organ is no longer able to resist the biomechanical forces that stress it. Traditionally, athlete has been viewed as a mere injury container and the injury itself as a broken piece that should be fixed up. Despite of such outlook, psychological research has shown athletes play an active role on the process of becoming injured and several psychosocial variables might influence on such. According to the seminal Andersen and Williams (1988, Williams and Andersen, 1998) model, the key psychological factor related to sport injury occurrence is the stress response. The present paper focuses on the preinjury phase, reviewing the concept of stress and analyzing the mechanisms involved in

* Corresponding author: Ass. Prof. Aurelio Olmedilla. Dpt. Personality, Assessment and Psychological Treatments. University of Murcia. 30100 Murcia (Spain). E-mail: olmedilla@um.es.

sport injury occurrence. It also reviews the experiences of interventions aimed to cope with stress and the empirical evidence of such interventions preventing sport injuries.

The Beginnings of the Study of the Stress-Sport Injury Relationships

The interest in psychological factors affecting sport injuries dates back to the 1970's when several authors tried to find relationships between personality traits and injury vulnerability (see, for instance, Williams and Andersen, 2007). However, such attempts, some of which found differences between injured and non-injured athletes, while others did not (see Andersen and Williams, 1988), brought about a more interactional approach (see Fischer, 1984, for a claim of a Person x Situation outlook instead of the static trait approach) where the concept of stress caught the attention of researchers.

By the seventies, stress had already been shown to play a role in disease promotion (see Krantz, Glass, Contrada and Miller, 1981) and accident occurrence in the work setting (see Burham's 2009 review). In this way, Holmes, in 1970 (cited in Andersen and Williams, 1988), having recently developed the Social Readjustment Rating Scale for assessing stressful life events with his colleague Rahe (Holmes and Rahe, 1967), found that there was a greater likelihood for football players to become injured when they had experienced important life events. This was the first of a series of studies that, in many cases, found greater incidence of sport injuries when athletes were exposed to high stress levels (Bramwell, Masuda, Wagner, and Holmes, 1975; Coddington and Troxell, 1980; Cryan and Alles, 1983; Lysens, Auweele, and Ostyn, 1986; Passer and Seese, 1983). These and some other results led Andersen and Williams (1988) to propose a model that aimed to provide a theoretical framework for explaining the relationship between stress and other psychosocial factors and injury outcome.

The Andersen and Williams's Stress and Injury Model

The Andersen and Williams's (1988) model, slightly revised years later (Williams and Andersen, 1998), is centered on the stress response, bidirectionaly related to the athlete's cognitive appraisal of a potentially stressful situation and the physiological and cognitive aspects of the stress response. As Williams and Andersen (1998, 2007) pointed out, the athlete makes an appraisal of the sport demands, the adequacy of his/hers resources for coping with the demands, and the consequences of meeting or failing to meet them. Cognitive appraisal triggers the physiological and attentional aspects of the stress response. Likewise, such changes influence cognitive appraisal in a bidirectional way.

In turn, stress response is influenced by three major factors: personality, history of stressors, and coping resources. According to the authors, the athlete's history of stressors (previous injuries, life events, daily hassles) influences the stress response by means of the cognitive appraisal of the situation and/or the physiological and attentional changes that are provoked.

In the same way, personality factors such as locus of control, sense of coherence, hardiness, trait anxiety and achievement motivation can directly affect to the stress response, or either a) moderate the influence of the history of stressors or b) are shaped by such previous stressors in the idiosyncratic way the individual cope with them. Finally, coping resources (sleep patterns, nutritional habits, social support network, stress management skills, etc.) act on the stress response either directly or by moderating the influence of previous stressors (Williams and Andersen, 1998; 2007). Furthermore, the revised version of the model also included a bidirectional relationship between coping resources and personality, highlighting the complex influences between the variables involved and the injury outcomes.

In the end, the model also includes the implementation of interventions aimed at reducing the stress response by both changing cognitive appraisals of potentially stressful events and modifying the physiological and attentional facets of the stress response involved in the sport injury.

Mechanisms Underlying the Stress-Injury Relationships

Rather than establishing a mere path of relationships between different psychosocial factors and injury outcomes, more or less based on empirical correlational studies, Andersen and Williams (1988, Williams and Andersen, 1998) hypothesized specific mechanisms involved in the stress-injury relationship. According to their model, on the one hand, stress response increases generalized muscle tension that can lead to a motor coordination disturbance as well as a reduction in flexibility and an increase in fatigue. On the other hand, stress response might affect the attention narrowing of the visual field, responsible for the lack of noticing relevant peripheral information and increased distractibility.

Muscle Tension

There are a broad number of studies that have shown the role of stress in increasing muscle tension, leading to diseases such as headaches or musculoskeletal disorders (Lundberg et al., 1999). Nevertheless, no one from the sport psychology field has directly explored the relationships between stress reactivity in terms of muscle tension and injury outcomes. There is just indirect evidence concerning such a relationship. For instance, Hicks, Inman, Deharo, and Hicks (1999) found that the consistency of hand use, considered as a measure of motor coordination, was related to sport injuries. More specifically, Arnason, Andersen, Holme, Engebretsen and Bahr (2008) showed that eccentric strength training with Nordic hamstring lowers, combined with warm-up stretching (but not solely flexibility training), appears to reduce the risk of hamstring strains.

Attention Deficit

Stress has been shown to affect the central nervous system in different ways. As early as 1970, Kopell, Wittner, Lunde, Warrick, and Edwards, (1970) found a significant decrease in individuals' event-related potentials (ERP) amplitudes to visual stimuli when injecting glucocorticoids, the hormones secreted under stress conditions. This ERP amplitude decrease, which has been further confirmed (see Lupien, Maheu, Tu, Fiocco, and Schramek, 2007, for a review), reflects a state of hypovigilance and is coherent with Andersen and Williams (1988) hypothesis.

There are just a bunch of studies from the field of sport psychology focused on attentional narrowing as a result of stress condition and injury outcome. Williams and Andersen (1997) found that athletes with high injury risk profile and higher negative life events scores, presented slower central vision reaction time when faced with a stressful lab test consisting of detecting cues in the central and peripheral fields of vision when performing a Stroop test. This reduced reaction time when facing a stressful condition was interpreted as a demonstration of distractibility and vigilance decrease when suffering more major life events. Moreover, Williams and Andersen (1997) also found the characteristic "visual tunnelling" effect (Dirkin, 1983) under stress: the group of participants with high life event scores showed significant higher peripheral narrowing compared to the group with low life event scores. These results were in line with findings previously obtained by the same group (Williams, Tonymon and Andersen, 1990, 1991) who also used a stressful lab task condition and found that high negative life events were related to greater peripheral narrowing during the stress condition, supporting the Andersen and Williams (1988) hypothesis about mechanisms involved in the stress-injury outcome relationship. However, some other mechanisms might also be involved.

Other Mechanisms

Athletes are active subjects in the injury process, committing or omitting actions that can lead to an injury (Almeida, Olmedilla, Rubio and Palou, 2014). In fact, anyone could intuitively assume that the more risk-taking behaviors showed (such as competing when experiencing muscle aches, diving to head the ball among the defense or playing aggressively against the opponents), the greater the risk of becoming injured (Rubio, Pujals, de la Vega, Aguado, Henández, 2014). The same could be said regarding omitting behaviors such as avoiding a correct warm-up prior to the sport activity or not wearing the required protection.

Does the stress response and/or its moderating factors affect the risk-taking behaviors shown by the athletes? Petrie (1993) found that athletes who reported high levels of social support were at a higher risk of experiencing an injury, contrary to what would be expected. The author hypothesized that, under lower stress, high social support may provide a sense of confidence, which might provoke an athlete's risk-taking behaviors.

Stress has shown to negatively affect decision making, increasing riskier behaviour (for instance, altering reward-punishing sensitivity, see Starcke and Brand, 2012). Moreover, experimental studies have shown that elevated levels of stress-evoked glucocorticoid concentrations (typically related to chronic stress) increase riskier behaviors, the opposite effect of that experienced when a moderate increase in catecholamimes occurs (usually in cases of acute/moderate stress) thereby enhancing decision-making performance (Pabst, Brand, and Wolf, 2013).

Furthermore, even though there are no specific studies from the sport psychology field, the literature regarding the role of emotions in decision making and inducing riskier behaviors could shed light on the stress-injury relationship and the role of other mechanisms beyond attentional and coordination-flexibility factors. For instance, social stress has been related to risk-prone activities such as aggression and novelty seeking in response to impulsive decision-making (Reynolds, Schreiber, Geisel, MacPherson, Ernst and Lejuez, 2013), and the potentially stressful athletic situation involved in the Andersen and Williams's model has many connotations of a social stress. Likewise, negative affective states such as fear, disgust or anger directly influence risk-taking behavior (Bodenhausen, 1993). It is assumed that such an influence is due to the fact that when under stress either a) cognitive resources are used for emotion regulation and are thereby distracted from inhibitory processes that might control risky behaviors (Baumeister, Vohs and Tice, 2007), or b) risk engagement reduces distress (Baker, Piper, McCarthy, Majeskie and Fiore, 2004).

Regardless of the explanation, scientific literature has shown that people under stress conditions have difficulty in regulating the focus of their attention, memory and psychomotor processes (McEwan, 2006) as well as in making decisions, and show an increasein risk-taking behaviors (Reynolds et al., 2013) that could result in sport injury.

Preventing Sport Injuries through Stress Control Strategies

According to the Andersen and Williams's model (1988) and its further review (Williams and Andersen, 1998), the stress is a key factor in the pathogenesis of a sport injury (Dunn, Smith, and Smoll, 2001; Galambos, Terry, Moyle, and Locke, 2005; Hanton, Fletcher, and Coughlan, 2005; Johnson and Ivarsson, 2011). Thus, from a psychological perspective, stress control might be a basic strategy for a sport injury prevention program. Nevertheless, there are just a few studies that have attempted to test the effectiveness of psychological programs in preventing sport injuries. Moreover, the empirical data shows controversial results. Such discrepancies have been attributed to different factors, such as the use of very reduced

(Tranaeus, Johnson, Engstrom, Skillgate, and Werner, 2014) or heterogeneous samples (for instance, combining male and females, see Edvardsson, Ivarsson, and Johnson, 2012) without considering the stress reactivity differences.

Additionally, there is a lack of clinical assay control and isolation of the components of the programs, using different techniques for training stress control management, as well as other psychological intervention strategies (see Johnson, Tranaeus, and Ivarsson, 2014).

The next section provides a review of the characteristics and results of studies that have tested the effectiveness of psychological intervention programs for reducing sport injury.

Psychological Intervention Programs for Reduction of Injury: An Overview

A literature review revealed that just only 14 studies have tested the effectiveness of psychological interventions in reducing sport injuries. Three out of these 14 are not focused on sport injury prevention but are general mental training programs that have also tested their effect on in sport injury incidence (DeWitt, 1980; Fenker and Lambiotte, 1987; Murphy, 1988). Eleven of them are specifically aimed to prevent sport injuries based on stress management.

As can be seen in Table 1, the systematic testing of the effectiveness of psychological programs for preventing injuries started during the 1980's, though there has only been a clear increment in its number since the beginning of the present century.

Presented in a chronological order, a study by DeWitt (1980) showed a substantial decrease in reported injuries in varsity basketball and soccer players after a combination of cognitive techniques (mental rehearsal exercises aimed to control tension), muscle relaxation and physiological feedback training. Fenker and Lambiotte (1987) carried out a psychological intervention program aimed at controlling competitive and training stress with an American college football team though not specifically oriented to reduce injuries. The program included imagery-training techniques combined with a process-oriented approach to performance. They found an over 33% reduction in the number of injuries during the following two seasons compared to the previous one (from 18 to 12 and 13, respectively). Murphy (1988), refers the first time a sport psychologist was recruited by the US Olympic Committee for providing psychological services to the 1987 US Olympic Festival.

Table 1. Injury prevention intervention studies

Study	Population	N	Intervention	Intervention effects
DeWitt (1980)	Basketball, football players	18	Biofeedback	Reduced injuries
Fenker and Lambiotte (1987)	Major college football team	30	Relaxation/Imaginery	33% reduction
Murphy (1988)	Team athletes	12	Relaxation/Pain control	Reduced injuries
May and Brown (1989)	Olympic alpine skiers	18	Relaxation/Imaginery	Reduced injuries, increased self-confidence
Schomer (1990)	Marathon runners	10	Attentional strategies	Facilitated heavy training with injury
Davis (1991)	Collegiate swimmers and football players	21	Stress management	52% reduction in swimming injuries, 33% reduction in football injuries
Kerr y Goss (1996)	Elite gymnasts	24	Stress management	Reduced injuries and stress level
Perna et al. (1998)	Collegiate rowers	34	Cognitive behavioral Stress management	Reduced injuries and illness. Robust association but non-significant
Perna et al. (2003)	Collegiate rowers	40	Cognitive behavioral Stress management	Reduced injuries and illness
Kolt et al. (2004)	Elite gymnasts	20	Stress management	Reduced injuries, No statistically significant differences

Study	Population	N	Intervention	Intervention effects
Johnson et al. (2005)	Competitive soccer players	32	Stress management, critical incidence	Reduced injuries and stress level
Maddison and Prapavessis (2005)	Competitive male rugby players	38	Stress management, CMSM	Reduced injuries and stress level
Noh et al. (2007)	Female ballet dancers	45	Autogenic Training, Broad-based Coping Skills	Reduced injuries, frequency and time lost
Edvarsson et al. (2012)	Junior soccer players	29	Cognitive behavioral Biofeedback	No significant difference between the control and experimental group
Tranaeus et al. (2014)	Elite floorball players	401	Stress management	Reduced injuries, No statistically significant differences
Olmedilla et al. (in preparation)	Junior soccer players	112	Relaxation/Imaginery/ Setting Goals	No significant difference between the control and experimental group

He reported the results of the work with one of the teams that had 7 of 12 players injured (2 seriously), leaving not even enough healthy players to hold a game. He carried out relaxation training with the athletes and pain control techniques with some of them. After the psychological training, all of the athletes exhibited pain reduction and the 12 were able to compete. Still in the eighties, May and Brown (1989) used a multifaceted program including attentional shift, visualization, mental skills training, team building and communication skills training with the US Olympic skiing team prior to and during the Calgary Olympic Games. The authors found adecrease in injuries, as well as an increase in self-confidence and self-control. Schomer (1990) also found a relationship between associative thinking strategies in marathon runners and a decline in overload injuries, facilitating athletes' heavy training even when injured.

During the nineties, there were three studies aimed at investigating the effectiveness of psychological interventions in sport injury prevention. Davis

(1991), for instance, used a psychological intervention consisting of visualization and relaxation for stress management with collegiate swimmers and soccer players.

He found injuries had a remarkable decrease of 52% in swimmers and 33% in soccer players. Nevertheless, Kerr and Goss (1996) applied Meichenbaum's stress inoculation training during eight months to a group of 24 male and female elite gymnasts and even though findings indicate the stress management program did reduce athletes' stress levels and enabled them to cope with the frustration of minor injuries, there were no significant findings for the effect of stress management on injury prevention. Perna, Antoni, and Schneiderman (1998) founded a quite robust (d = .67), albeit non-significant, effect on injury reduction when they used a stress management program with a very small sample of collegiate rowers. To the contrary, the same group of researchers (Perna, Antoni, Baum, Gordon and Schneiderman, 2003), working in this case with a larger sample of varsity rowers found a statistically significant drop of injuries and illnesses of the group receiving a behavioral-cognitive stress management program compared to the group which did not received the intervention. Nevertheless, Kolt, Hume, Smith, and Williams (2004) failed to find significant differences between treatment and placebo groups when they used a stress-management program consisting of 12 one-hour sessions with 20 New Zealand elite gymnasts (half of them assigned to the treatment and half to the placebo group). Even though they recorded less injuries in the treatment group compared to the group that received only the anthropometric measures and lecturers on nutrition during the 9 month period following the intervention, these differences were not statistically significant.

Johnson, Ekengren and Andersen (2005), working with soccer players, carried out a study in which they took 32 athletes, previously identified to be at risk of injury according to their stress levels and other psychosocial factors involved, and assigned them to either a control or a intervention group consisted of training in six mental skills (somatic and cognitive relaxation, stress management skills, goal-setting skills, attribution and self-confidence training, and identification and discussion about critical incident related to sport and everyday life situations). Results showed a significant drop in both stress level and injury occurrence during the intervention period compared to the control group. Using the same paradigm, in this case with a sample of 470 rugby players, Maddison and Prapavessis (2005) carried out two related studies. In the first one they assessed history of stressors, coping strategies and social support in order to identify athletes at risk for suffering sport injuries, according to Andersen and Williams's model (1988, Williams and Andersen,

1998). Once they identified 48 players at risk, the second study consisted of a testing whether a cognitive behavioral stress management intervention program could be useful for reducing sport injuries. Their results showed athletes at risk showed a reduction in time missed due to injuries as well as stress levels compared to non-intervention counterparts.

Noh, Morris and Andersen (2007), in this case with 45 Korean dancers, tested the efficacy of an autogenic training program, a broad-based coping skills training program including autogenic training, imagery and self-talk, and a control group which did not received any specific psychological intervention. Authors found that dancers at the broad-based coping skills condition significantly shortened the average time elapsed since injury to dancer return compared to the control group.

However, other studies did not find significant differences. Edvarsson, et al. (2012) used a combined intervention including biofeedback training, somatic relaxation, thought stopping, emotions/problems focused coping, goal setting and keeping a critical incident diary in a sample of 29 junior soccer players and they could not find significant differences between control and treatment groups. Tranaeus et al. (2014) also failed to find statistically significant differences between a treatment group consisting of 11 soccer teams receiving a 6-session stress management program and a control group (12 soccer teams which did not received any specific psychological intervention). Finally, Olmedilla, Rubio, Ortega and Boladeras (in preparation) also did not find significant differences when 6 junior soccer teams receiving an intervention including relaxation, goal-setting, stress management, and visualization, were compared to a control group consisted of 2 other junior soccer teams.

Proposals for Future Research

As was previously mentioned, the empirical evidence on the effectiveness of psychological interventions focused on stress management, with or without some other facets, is far from being established. If there is no statistically significant reduction in sport injuries compared to some other group or regarding the previous history of injuries, does it refute the Andersen and Williams's model? Does it mean intervention programs are not properly designed or applied? Are there non-controlled variables affecting the results obtained? Is this a matter of inadequacy of experimental designs or assessment procedures?

Firstly, it should be stated that Andersen and Williams's model itself pointed out the multidetermined nature of the phenomenon. Moreover, the implementation of programs such as those reviewed should include many aspects, such as the number of effective sessions the athletes receive, the character of standardized interventions regardless the reactivity to stress of each individual and his/her idiosyncratic factors, etc. Moreover, the length of the interventions and the preservation of the achievements are another issue that should be taken into account. Most of the studies have been designed to be applied short term and almost no one has continued research for more than one season to show how long the gains are preserved and how they influence sport injuries (Finch, 2006). For that reason, further research should be carried out in order to test the effectiveness of psychological intervention programs on the prevention of sport injuries.

In this line, Almeida et al. (2014), based on the *Global Psychological Approach to Sport Injuries* and its three proposal axes (causal, temporal, and conceptual, see Olmedilla and García-Mas, 2009), highlight the need for integrating the different collections of empirical data, as well as to agree on what a sport injury is, to what extent it is measured though the outcomes typically used and how the relationships between psychological factors and sport injury should be methodologically studied.

Likewise, Johnson (2007) emphasizes the need for clarification and agreement regarding two basic aspects: theoretical background and research designs, assessment instruments and statistical tests. Concerning the theoretical issues, Andersen and Williams's (1988) model is useful for pointing out the role of several psychological factors and the sport injury. However, some other approaches could contribute to a more comprehensive perspective, such as the Hanin's (2000) Individual Zones of Optimal Functioning (IZOF) model. Several studies have shown that it can be used as a theoretical background for detecting emotional antecedents which have shown to be related to sport injuries (Devonport, Lane, and Hall, 2003; Mårtensson, 2004; Olmedilla, Ortega and Gómez, 2014).

Regarding research, assessment and statistical analyses, future research should insist on controlled trials with larger samples, comparing treatments, as well as using non-treatment groups. Moreover, although not devoid of difficulties (Johnson, 2007), longitudinal studies are necessary in order to test the dynamic aspects involved, and prospective, instead of retrospective, gathering might protect against several biases the quality of the data (Almeida et al., 2014; Johnson et al., 2014). In this line, there are several concerns about the near to exclusive use of self-reports for assessing the relevant dimensions and collecting information. Effort should be made towards the introduction of task-based assessment, observational techniques, physiological and biochemical outcomes, as well as the promotion of new IT-based technologies in order to provide more accurate and multiplist data collection (Almeida et al., 2014). Likewise, statistical models based on general linear modelling would probably leave out relevant data (Johnson et al., 2014). Therefore, analyses based on latent growth curves, Bayesian analysis and structural equation modelling for testing changes might contribute to a more precise examination of the complex interactions between the independent variables (García-Mas, Pujals, Fuster-Parra, Nuñez, and Rubio, 2014; Johnson et al., 2014). Likewise, qualitative studies can also contribute to a better comprehension of the role of psychological factors in sport injury and its prediction and prevention, as a few studies have shown (Georgiadis, Biddle and Auweele, 2001; Johnson, 2011).

Furthermore, as Johnson and colleagues have pointed out (Johnson et al., 2014; Tranaeus et al., 2014) several aspects should be considered when testing the preventive efficacy of psychological interventions: a clear definition of the type of injury (overload vs. traumatic injuries; self-produced vs. sustained by opponent collision), age, gender, competitive level and position, as well as cultural issues that could be involved. Finally, staff participation and engagement can make the difference between successful and unsuccessful interventions in terms of reaching the preventive goal (Tranaeus et al., 2014).

References

Almeida, P., Olmedilla, A., Rubio, V. J., and Palou, P. (2014). Psychology in the realm of sport injury: What it is all about. *Revista de Psicología del Deporte*, 23(2), 395-400.

Andersen, M. B. and Williams, J. M. (1988). A model of stress and athletic injury: Prediction and prevention. *Journal of Sport and Exercise Psychology*, 10(3), 294-306.

Arnason, A., Andersen, T. E., Holme, I., Engebretsen, L., and Bahr, R. (2008). Prevention of hamstring strains in elite soccer: an intervention study. *Scandinavian Journal of Medicine and Science in Sports*, 18(1), 40-48.

Baker, T. B., Piper, M. E., McCarthy, D. E., Majeskie, M. R., and Fiore, M. C. (2004). Addiction motivation reformulated: an affective processing model of negative reinforcement. *Psychological Review*, 111(1), 33-51.

Baumeister, R. F., Vohs, K. D. and Tice, D. M. (2007). The strength model of self-control. *Current Directions in Psychological Science*, 16(6), 351-355.

Bodenhausen, G. V. (1993). Emotions, arousal, and stereotypic judgments: A heuristic model of affect and stereotyping. In: D. M. Mackie and D. L. Hamilton (Eds.), *Affect, cognition, and stereotyping: Interactive processes in group perception* (pp. 13-37). San Diego, CA: Academic Press.

Bramwell, S. T., Masuda, M., Wagner, N. N., and Holmes, T. H. (1975). Psychological factors in athletic injuries: Development and application of the Social and Athletic Readjustment Rating Scale (SAARS). *Journal of Human Stress*, 1(1), 6-20.

Burnham, J. C., 2009. *Accident Prone: A History of Technology, Psychology, and Misfits of the Machine Age.* Chicago: The University of Chicago Press.

Coddington, R. D. and Troxell, J. R. (1980). The effect of emotional factors on football injury rates: A pilot study. *Journal of Human Stress*, 6(1), 3-5.

Cryan, P. O. and Alles, E. F. (1983). The relationships between stress and football injuries. *Journal of Sports Medicine and Physical Illness*, 23(1), 52-58.

Davis, J. O. (1991). Sport injuries and stress management. An opportunity for research. *The Sport Psychologist,* 5(2), 175-182.

Devonport, T. J., Lane, A. M. and Hall, R. J. (2003, July). Affective state profile of athletes prior to best, worst and injured performance. *Paper presented at 8th Annual Congress of the European College of Sport Science*, Salzburg, Austria.

DeWitt, D. J. (1980). Cognitive and biofeedback training for stress reduction with university athletes. *Journal of Sport Psychology,* 2, 288-294.

Dirkin, G. R. (1983). Cognitive tunnelling: Use of visual information under stress. *Perceptual and Motor Skills*, 56(1), 191-198.

Dunn, E., Smith, R. and Smoll, F. (2001). Do sport-specific stressors predict athletic injury?. *Journal of Science and Medicine in Sport,* 4(3), 283-291.

Edvardsson, A., Ivarsson, A. and Johnson, U. (2012). Is a cognitive-behavioural biofeedback intervention useful to reduce injury risk in junior football players?. *Journal of Sports Science and Medicine,* 11(2), 331-338.

Fenker, R. and Lambiotte, J. (1987). A performance enhancement program for a college football team: One incredible season. *The Sport Psychologist,* 1(3), 224-236.

Finch, C. (2006). A new framework for research leading to sports injury prevention. *Journal of Science and Medicine in Sport,* 9(1-2), 3-9.

Fischer, A. C. (1984). New directions in sport personality research. In: J. M. Silva and R. S. Weinberg (Eds.). *Psychological foundations of sport* (pp. 70-80). Champaign, IL: Human Kinetics.

Galambos, S., Terry, P., Moyle, G., and Locke, S. (2005). Psychological predictors of injury among elite athletes. *British Journal of Sports Medicine,* 39(6), 351-354.

García-Mas, A., Pujals, C., Fuster,-Parra, P., Núñez, A., and Rubio, V. (2014). Determinación de las variables psicológicas y deportivas relevantes a las lesiones deportivas: Un análisis bayesiano [Determination of the psychological and sportive variables related to sports injuries: a bayesian analysis]. *Revista de Psicología del Deporte,* 23(2), 423-429.

Georgiadis, M., Biddle, S. J. H. and Auweele, Y. V. (2001). Cognitive, emotional, and behavioral connotations of task and ego goal orientation profiles: An ideographic approach using hierarchical class analysis. *International Journal of Sport Psychology,* 32 (1), 1-20.

Hanin, Y. L. (2000). *Emotions in Sport*. Human Kinetics, Champaign.

Hanton, S., Fletcher, D. and Coughlan, G. (2005). Stress in elite sport performers: a comparative study of competitive and organizational stressors. *Journal of Sports Sciences,* 23(10), 1129-1141.

Hicks, R. A., Inman, G., Deharo, D., and Hicks, G. J. (1999). Consistency of hand use, exercise, and sports-related injuries. *Perceptual and Motor Skills*, 88(3), 1359-1360.

Holmes, T. H. and Rahe, R. H. (1967). The Social Readjustment Rating Scale. *Journal of Psychosomatic Research*, 11(2), 213-218.

Johnson, U. (2007). Psychosocial antecedents of sport injury, prevention, and intervention: an overview of theoretical approaches and empirical findings. *International Journal of Sport and Exercise Psychology,* 5(4), 352-369.

Johnson, U. (2011). Athletes' experiences of psychosocial risk factors preceding injury. *Qualitative Research in Sport, Exercise and Health*, 3(1), 99-115.

Johnson, U., Ekengren, J. and Andersen, M. B. (2005). Injury prevention in Sweden: Helping soccer player at risk. *Journal of Sport and Exercise Psychology,* 27(1), 32-38.

Johnson, U. and Ivarsson, A. (2011) Psychological predictors of sport injuries among junior soccer players. *Scandinavian Journal of Medicine and Science in Sports,* 21(1), 129-136.

Johnson, U., Tranaeus, U. and Ivarsson, A. (2014). Current status and future challenges in psychological research of sport injury prediction and prevention: A methodological perspective. *Revista de Psicología del Deporte,* 23(2), 401-409.

Kerr, G. and Goss, J. (1996). The effects and stress management program on injuries and stress level. *Journal of Applied Sport Psychology,* 8(1), 109-117.

Kolt, G., Hume, P. A., Smith, P., and Williams, M. (2004). Effects of a stress-management program on injury and stress of competitive gymnasts. *Perceptual and Motor Skills,* 99 (1), 195-207.

Kopell, B. S., Wittner, W. K., Lunde, D., Warrick, G., and Edwards, D. (1970). Cortisol effects on averaged evoked potentials, alpha-rhythm, time estimation, and two-flash fusion threshold. *Psychosomatic Medicine*, 32(1), 39-49.

Krantz, D. S., Glass, D. C., Contrada, R. J., and Miller, N. E. (1981). Behavior and Health. *The National Science Foundation: Five year outlook on science and technology: 1981 Source materials* (Vol. 2, pp. 561-588). Washington, D.C.; Government Printing Office.

Lundberg, U., Dohns, I. E., Melin, B., Sandsjö, L., Palmerud, G., Kadefors, R., Ekstrom, M., and Parr, D. (1999). Psychophysiological stress responses, muscle tension, and neck and shoulder pain among supermarket cashiers. *Journal of Occupational Health Psychology*, 4(3), 245-255.

Lupien, S. J., Maheu, F., Tu, M., Fiocco, A., and Schramek, T. E. (2007). The effects of stress and stress hormones on human cognition: Implications for the field of brain and cognition. *Brain and Cognition*, 65(3), 209-237.

Lysens, R., Auweele, Y. V. and Ostyn, M. (1986). The relationshps between psychosocial factors and sport injuries. *Journal of Sports Medicine and Physical Fitness*, 26(1), 77-84.

Maddison, R. and Prapavessis, H. (2005). A psychological approach to the prediction and prevention of athletic injury. *Journal of Sport and Exercise Psychology,* 27(3), 289-310.

Mårtensson, C. M. (2004). *A study about the relationship between performance related emotional state and the risk of sustaining athletic injuries of speedway drivers at elite level.* Unpublished Master's dissertation, School of Social and Health Science, Halmstad University, Sweden.

May, J. R. and Brown, L. (1989). Delivery of psychological service to the US Alpine ski team prior to and during the Olympics in Calgary. *The Sport Psychologist,* 3(4), 320-329.

McEwen, B. S. (2006). Protective and damaging effects of stress mediators: central role of the brain. *Dialogues in Clinical Neuroscience*, 8(4), 367-382.

Murphy, S. M. (1988). The on-site provision of sport psychology service at the US Olympic Festival. *The Sport Psychologist,* 2(4), 337-350.

Noh, Y. E., Morris, T. and Andersen, M. B. (2007). Psychological intervention for reduction of injury in ballet dancers. *Research in Sports Medicine,* 15(1), 13-32.

Olmedilla, A. and García-Mas, A. (2009). El Modelo Global Psicológico de las Lesiones Deportivas. *Acción Psicológica*, 6(2), 77-91.

Olmedilla, A., Ortega, E. and Gómez, J. M. (2014). Influencia de la lesión deportiva en los cambios del estado de ánimo y de la ansiedad precompetitiva en futbolistas [Influence of sport injury on mood states and competitive anxiety in soccer players]. *Cuadernos de Psicología del Deporte,* 14(1), 9-10.

Olmedilla, A., Rubio, V., Ortega, E., and Boladeras, A. (in preparation). *Preventing sport injuries: A psychological intervention over Spanish soccer youth players*.

Pabst, S., Brand, M. and Wolf, O. T. (2013). Stress and decision making: A few minutes make all the difference. *Behavioural Brain Research*, 250, 39-45.

Passer, M. W. and Seese, M. D. (1983). Life stress and athletic injury: Examination of positive versus negative events and three moderator variables. *Journal of Human Stress*, 9(1), 11-16.

Perna, F. M., Antoni, M. and Schneiderman, N. (1998). Psychological intervention prevents injury/illness among athletes [Abstract]. *Journal of Applied Sport Psychology,* 10 (Suppl.), 53-54.

Perna, F. M., Antoni, M. H., Baum, A., Gordon, P., and Schneiderman, N. (2003). Cognitive behavioral stress management effects on injury and illness among competitive athletes: a randomized clinical trial. *Annals of Behavioral Medicine,* 25(1), 66-73.

Petrie, T. A. (1993). The moderating effects of social support and playing status on the life stress-injury relationship. *Journal of Applied Sport Psychology*, 5(1), 1-16.

Reynolds, E. K., Schreiber, W. M., Geisel, K., MacPherson, L., Ernst, M., and Lejuez, C. W. (2013). Influence of social stress on risk-taking behavior in adolescents. *Journal of Anxiety Disorders*, 27(3), 272-277.

Rubio, V. J., Pujals, C., de la Vega, R., Aguado, D., and Hernández, J. M. (2014). Autoeficacia y lesions deportivas: ¿factor protector o de riesgo?

[Self-efficacy and sport injuries: Is this a risk or a protective factor?]. *Revista de Psicología del Deporte*, 23(2), 439-444.

Schomer, H. H. (1990). A cognitive strategy training program for marathon runners: Ten case studies. *South African Journal of Research in Sport, Physical Education and Recreation,* 13, 47-78.

Starcke, K. and Brand, M. (2012). Decision making under stress: a selective review. *Neuroscience and Biobehavioral Reviews*, 36(4), 1228-1248.

Tranaeus, U., Johnson, U., Engstrom, B., Skillgate, E., and Werner, S. (2014). A psychological injury prevention group intervention in Swedish floorball. *Knee Surgery, Sports Traumatology, Arthroscopy.* doi: 10.1007/s00167-014-3133-z.

Williams, J. M. and Andersen, M. B. (1997). Psychosocial lnfluences on Central and Peripheral vision and reaction time during demandin tasks. *Behavioral Medicine*, 22(4), 160-167.

Williams, J. M. and Andersen, M. B. (1998). Psychosocial antecedents of sport injury: Review and critique of the stress and injury model. *Journal of Applied Sport Psychology*, 10(1), 5-25.

Williams, J. M. and Andersen, M. B. (2007). Psychosocial antecedents of sport injury and interventions for risk reduction. In: G. Tenenbaum and R. C. Eklund (Eds.), *Handbook of sport psychology* (pp. 379-403). New York: John Willey.

Williams, J. M., Tonymon, P. and Andersen, M. B. (1990). Effects of life event stress on anxiety and peripheral narrowing. *Behavioral Medicine*, 16(4), 174-181.

Williams, J. M., Tonymon, P. and Andersen, M. B. (1991). Effects of stressors and coping resources on anxiety and preripheral narrowing in recreational athletes. *Journal of Applied Sport Psychology*, 3(2), 126-141.

In: Sports Injuries
Editor: Gabrielle Hopkins
ISBN: 978-1-63463-305-5

Chapter 5

INJURIES IN HURLING AND CAMOGIE: A REVIEW OF INCIDENCE, MANAGEMENT AND PREVENTION

Edel Marie Quinn*
Specialist Registrar in Surgery,
Royal College of Surgeons in Ireland, Ireland

ABSTRACT

Background: Hurling, and its female equivalent, camogie, are Irish field sports played with a stick called a hurley and a ball called a sliotar. Both sports have some similarities to field hockey and the Scottish sport of shinty. Hurling is a contact sport and various associated injury patterns have been recognised. Players can use personal protective equipment in the form of helmets, handguards, mouthguards and shinguards. As of 2010, wearing of a helmet with a faceguard is mandatory for all players during both training and match play.

Injury Patterns: A study of attendances at an Irish emergency department showed that 12.3% of orthopaedic presentations were sports related; in another study 41% of sports related injuries were due to hurling. The most common injuries now encountered are hand injuries, although head injuries are also common. Serious head, facial and eye injuries have been reported and permanent visual deficits have been

* Contact: Edel Marie Quinn, Department of Surgery, University Hospital Waterford, Telephone: 0035351 84800, Email: edelquinn@rcsi.ie

sustained. Injuries to the external ear, spine, teeth and muscular injuries have also all been described.

Injury Prevention: It has been shown that head injuries are more common in players not wearing helmets. Introduction of helmets with faceguards has dramatically reduced the incidence of head trauma. Hurling related facial fractures halved over a 20 year period following introduction of voluntary helmet use and a significant reduction in eye injury rates was seen in adolescents following introduction of mandatory helmet wearing. However, current helmet design does not protect the external ear and players are not entirely satisfied with the helmet performance. With reductions in head injury rates, hand injury has become more common. In fact, a recent study has shown an association between helmet wearing and hand injury. The majority of hurling and camogie players have tried using commercially available handguards but <5% of players regularly use them. The majority of hand fractures occur in players not wearing any hand protection.

Conclusions: In summary, hurling and camogie related trauma is common and can be significant. Use of protective equipment has been shown to reduce head and facial injuries. However, hand trauma remains a significant problem, requiring development of better, more acceptable preventive strategies.

BACKGROUND

Hurling, and its female equivalent, camogie, are Irish field sports played with an ash stick called a hurley and a leather covered ball called a sliotar. Teams are composed of fifteen players who are allowed to both handle the ball (Figure 1a) as well as play the ball with the hurley (Figure 1b). There is close contact between players. [1] Hurling is known for its speed, skill and ferocity, and remains an amateur sport regulated by the Gaelic Athletic Association (GAA). [2] It is a sport predominantly played at a young age, with few players over the age of 40 years.

The standard hurling pitch is 135–145 m long and 80–90 m wide and has a goal at each end composed of two posts, which are set 6.4 m apart, and connected above the ground by a crossbar set at a height of 2.5 m. A ball hit over the bar is worth one point. A ball that is hit under the bar is called a goal and is worth three points. [3] A good strike with a hurley can propel the ball up to 150km/h, and to a distance of more than 80m. [4] The sport has some similarities to the sports of field hockey, lacrosse and the Scottish sport of shinty. [5] However, hurling differs from field hockey and lacrosse in that the sliotar can be caught in the hand and carried for not more than four steps, then struck in the air or struck on the ground with the hurley; the ball can also be kicked or slapped with an open hand (the hand pass) for short-range passing [3].

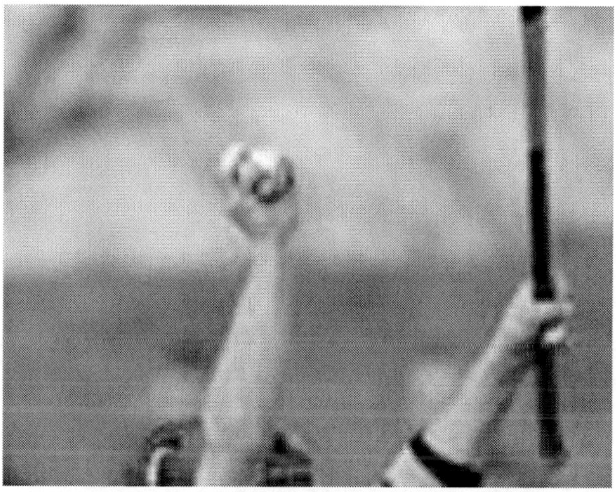

(a)

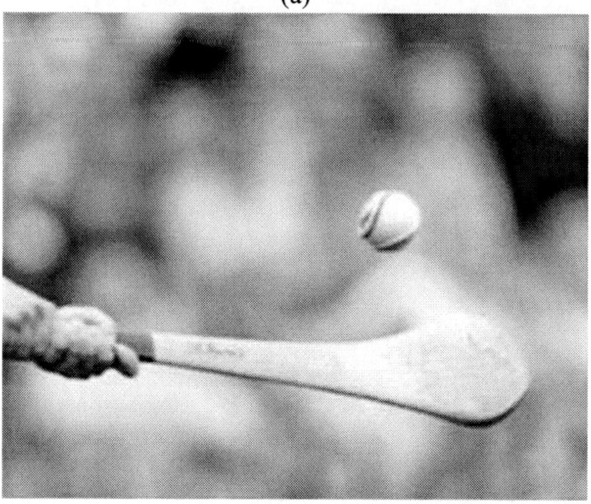

(b)

Figure 1. Hurling is played with a ball called a sliotar and a stick called a hurley; (a) The sliotar can be caught and played with the hand; (b) alternatively the sliotar can also be raised and hit using the hurley.

While a national sport of Ireland, hurling is also played worldwide among members of the Irish diaspora in the United States, Canada, Australia, New Zealand, Europe, South Africa and Argentina. [6] Hurling is played throughout Ireland but has its highest percentage of players in the south of the country where players are serviced by hospitals in Cork, Kilkenny, Waterford and Limerick, as well as the capital city Dublin (Figure 2).

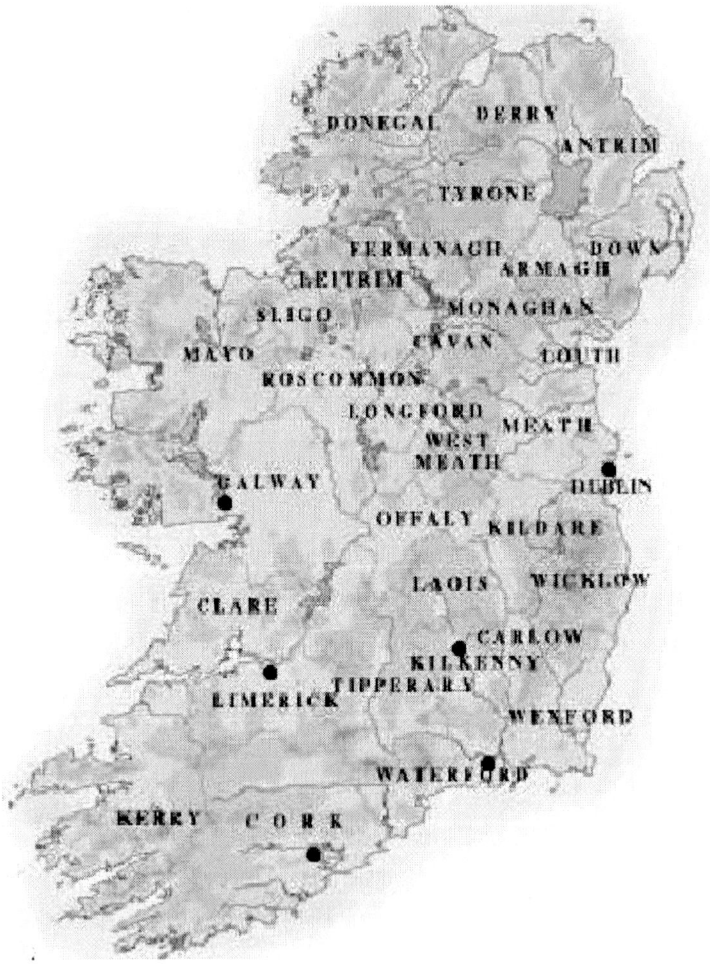

Figure 2. Map of Ireland with black dots representing locations of hospitals serving majority of hurling and camogie related injuries.

The unrestricted height swing of the hurley, which typically weighs 0.6kg and measures up to 1 metre in length, and the cricket-ball like nature of the sliotar mean that injury is an ever present risk in hurling. [7] Therefore, some personal protective equipment is available for players, namely helmets with faceguards, handguards, mouthguards and shinguards. Up until 2010 wearing of any protective equipment was purely player choice. However, since then it has been mandatory for all players to wear a helmet with faceguard during training and competitive matches [7].

Injury Rates and Demographics

A number of studies have attempted to record the frequency of injuries sustained playing hurling and camogie. Watson followed 74 players prospectively for one season and found they averaged 4.3 hours of training and 1.15 hours of matches per week. [8] There were 92 match and 43 training related injuries; a total of 342 injuries per 10,000 hours of match play and 43 injuries per 10,000 hours of training. Injuries resulted in a mean time of 1.2 days in hospital, 20.3 days off sport and 13.3 days of restricted activity [8].

In a survey of two senior county hurling panels (the most elite hurlers, who play competitively to represent their county), 39 of 45 players (86.7%) received injuries to the head and face during their careers that have required suturing. [9] Four players (10.3%) reported such injuries as occurring more than 10 times, with 9 players (23.1%) experiencing such injuries between 5 and 10 times. Fourteen players (31.1%) out of the total of 45 players questioned, received what they would term as a serious eye injury. None of the study participants reported any degree of permanent vision loss following injury. However, forty-three players (95.6%) are aware of at least one player who has lost vision due to a serious eye injury during their career [9].

A survey of hurlers attending the emergency department with hurling related injuires found that most patients had already suffered at least one injury in the past (n=116, 71.2%); two-thirds of patients had between one and five previous injuries (n=108, 66.3%) and eight patients (4.9%) had more than six previous injuries. [3] A week or more of play was lost by 152 (93.3%) of those injured, whereas 89 (54.6%) lost more than 4 weeks. Owing to their injuries, 71 (43.6%) people missed work [3].

A survey of 139 active camogie players found that 37% (52 players) reported at least one injury requiring medical attention as a direct result of playing camogie in the preceding 12 months.[10] Twenty-seven players (19%)

reported more than one injury. Forty-six of 52 injured players (88%) sustained injury significant enough to impact on ability to play, requiring time out from camogie. Time out required from camogie was a mean of 24 days [10].

Most players affected by hurling and camogie injuries are young. A comprehensive study of 413 hurling related injuries found the age range of those injured to be 6-44 years. [11] The very young age profile was further emphasised in this study by documenting the age quartiles of all injured players, with the youngest 25% of players ranging from 6-14 years; the next 25% ranging from 15-18 years and a further 25% between 19 and 22 years. [11] This finding has been reinforced in other studies, such as that by Cuddihy in Kilkenny where half of all hurling and camogie related injuries occurred in the 15-25 year age group [12].

Injury Patterns

Hurling-related injuries have been studied and reported since the 1980s. Since those first studies, the pattern of injuries seen has changed in line with changes in both availability of and mandatory requirements to wear protective equipment. The most common injuries now encountered are hand injuries, [1,3,10,13] although head injuries also remain common. [14] Serious head, facial and eye injuries have been reported. [4,1516,17,18] and permanent visual deficits have been sustained. [4] Injuries to the external ear, [2] spine [19], teeth [15] and muscular injuries[8] have also all been described. Eight point seven percent of orthopaedic hospital admissions have been attributed to sports related injury. [20] In hurling counties in Ireland, up to 41% of sports related injuries have been attributed to hurling [12].

Earliest Studies

The earliest studies of hurling related injuries were descriptive in nature. A 1984 study of hurling and camogie injuries found that of 817 hurlers/camogie players attending hospital with injuries that year, hand injuries accounted for 36% and face and head injuries combined accounted for 28% of all presentations. [1] 90% of injured players were male, with an average age of 21 years; the average female age was 17.9 years. Similar findings of high hand and head injury rates were replicated in a study performed between 1987 and 1988. [12] Forty percent (n=350) of 864 sports-related injuries studied over the course of one year at a single emergency department were due to hurling and 4% (n=32) were sustained playing camogie. Hurling and camogie together accounted for over 70% of all sports related head, face and neck injuries and 55% of all hand and wrist injuries. Facial fractures were also common in the early reports. Carroll et al. reviewed 332 patients seen with facial fractures during the year 1993 and found 110 (33%) to be sports related. [21] Of these, the sports of Gaelic football (29), hurling (23), and camogie (2) accounted for almost half of sports related facial fractures. [21] It was clear that head, face and hand injuries were common occurrences in hurling and camogie. By the mid-1990s further studies were undertaken to assess means of prevention of these hurling related injuries. All patients treated for hurling related injuries at Cork Regional Hospital over the 12 month period from the 1st July 1992 to the 30th June 1993 were identified in a study by Crowley et al. [11] A total of 413 hurling players were treated at the hospital during the study period. The distribution of injuries was again dominated by two main sites – hand and head. Over half (56%) of the incidents involved damage to a player's hand while a further one fifth (20%) consisted of head injuries. These are remotely followed by ankle (5%), knee (5 %), leg (3%), shoulder (3 %), foot (2%) and arm (2%). The authors were the first to then analyse these injury patterns further by comparing those who wore helmets versus those who didn't, as described below.

Early Studies of Equipment Benefit

Cuddihy first reported on use of protective equipment in hurling and camogie in that study performed in 1987-1988. [12] In hurling and camogie only 45% and 30% respectively of those injured were wearing helmets. The relatively large number of facial as opposed to scalp injuries, was probably due to the fact that just under half of hurlers wore helmets to protect the scalp area but only one player was recorded as wearing both a faceguard and a helmet [12].

However, it was Crowley's study in 1993 which first clearly demonstrated statistical benefits of helmet use. [11] Information was noted regarding usage of helmets and faceguards for 346 (84%) of the 413 patients in their study. [11] Sixty-four percent of players were wearing a helmet at the time of their injury, while 44% of helmeted players also wore a faceguard. The distribution of site of injury for helmet users was compared with that for non-users and significant differences were seen between the two groups. Notably 41% of injuries suffered by non-helmet users involved the head compared with just 13% of helmet users - more than a three to one ratio. A further significant reduction in the rate of head injuries was seen in those wearing both helmets and faceguards with just 3% of players using 'helmet and faceguard' protection suffering from facial trauma compared with 21% of players using helmets only [11].

It was clear, at this stage, that head trauma was a significant, potentially preventable component of hurling related injury. However, other injuries are also frequently encountered and as helmet use became more common, the frequency of non-head injuries increased in importance.

Common Injury Sites

The distribution of injuries has evolved over time, along with developments in protective equipment use. As discussed, head and hand injuries together have always accounted for the highest proportion of injuries requiring hospital attendance – initially head injuries were the commonest injury site, however they have now been overtaken by hand injuries.

Head and Facial Injuries, Including Eye Injuries

Sports account for up to 29% of emergency department presentations with facial injuries. [18] In 864 sports related injuries treated at St Luke's Hopsital, Kilkenny in 1984, there were 113 lacerations to the head region sustained playing hurling compared to 26 in all other sports combined [12].

A study based in the Eye Department at Waterford Regional Hospital in 1995 [17] found 98 new eye injuries (of 5,835 new presentations) related to sport or sports equipment. Fifteen percent of injured patients were female and 85% male. Hurling and camogie together accounted for 30% of sports related eye injuries. The majority of injuries were due to a direct blow to the eye – 13 cases were struck by the ball, 13 by the hurley stick, 1 by a thumb, 1 by a kick, and 1 struck by the helmet of another player. Of twenty-nine players attending hospital with eye injuries sustained playing hurling/camogie, 9 patients were wearing an old style helmet without facemask which offers no face or eye protection, 7 were wearing no face, eye or head protection and one player took off an uncomfortable full helmet and facemask late in a game, and was subsequently injured [17].

A follow-up study of eye injuries at Waterford Regional Hospital was performed between 2003 and 2006. [4] During this study period, it became mandatory for players under the age of 18 to wear helmets with faceguards in all matches and training. [22] However, protective equipment use was still entirely optional for adult players. Sixty hurling-related eye injuries presented during the study period, with a male to female ratio of 58:2. Of these, 42 (70%) were the result of injury by the ball and 17 (28.3%) were the result of impact with the stick, whereas one injury resulted from collision with another player. Twenty-one (35%) players were wearing protective helmets at the time of injury. Of these, 15 were wearing helmets with an unmodified face mask, two were wearing helmets with a modified face mask and four were wearing a helmet without any face mask (Figure 3).

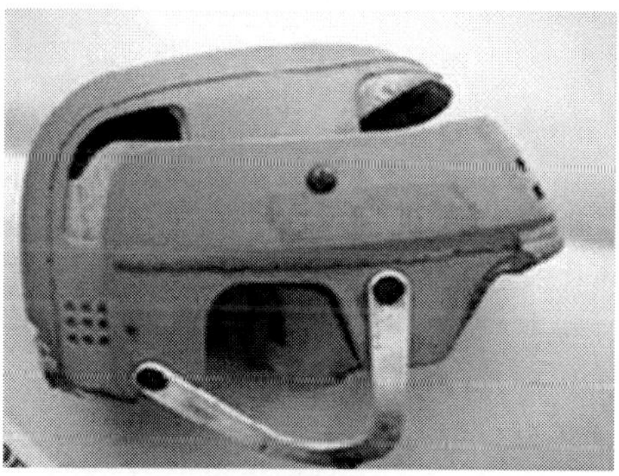

(a)

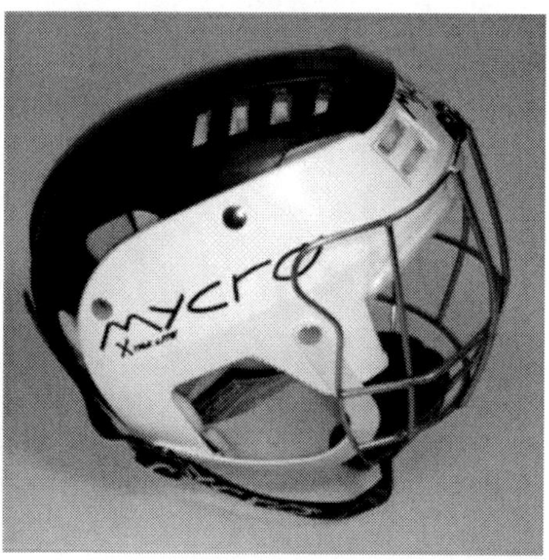

(b)

Figure 3. (a) Old style hurling helmet without faceguard (Cooper Ltd, Co Galway, Ireland); (b) newer design with full faceguard (Mycro Ltd, Cork, Ireland).

Sixteen (26.6%) hurling-related ocular injuries during this study period warranted hospitalisation. The average length of stay was 2.75 days, and nine patients required surgery including cataract removal, canalicular repair, scleral buckle for retinal dialysis, repair of macular hole, repair of lid laceration. Eleven injuries (18.3%) resulted in a permanent visual deficit [4].

A study of 70 hurling related facial injuries performed in 2007 found the majority (n=52) occurred in players wearing no helmet and only 18 occurred in those with a helmet. [15] Hurlers with no helmets sustained 32 facial lacerations, 10 facial fractures, 5 soft tissue injuries and 5 dental injuries. Hurlers wearing helmets sustained 6 facial lacerations, 5 facial fractures, 6 soft tissue injuries and 1 dental injury [15].

Hand Injuries

Hand injuries have always been prevalent in hurling and camogie. The early studies from the 1980s feature a large number of hand injuries especially fractures.[12] These mainly involved the first meta-carpal and proximal phalanx of thumb, the second mata-carpal and proximal phalanx of index finger and to a lesser extent the fifth metacarpal and proximal phalanx of the little finger (Figure 4). The mode of injury is invariably a direct blow from an opponent's hurley.

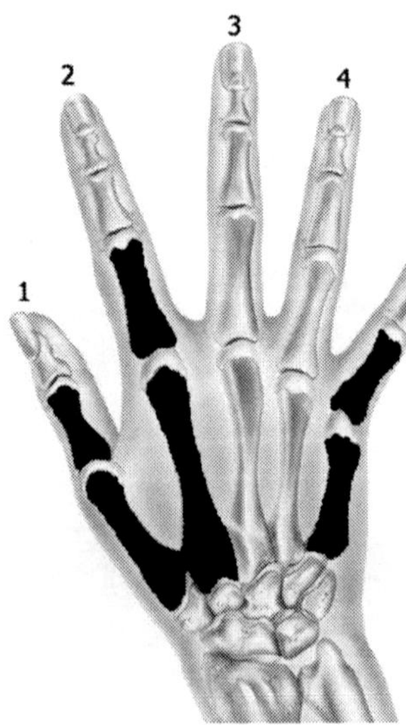

Figure 4. Most commonly encountered hand fractures: first metacarpal, proximal phalanx of thumb, second metacarpal and proximal phalanx of index finger and less commonly the fifth metacarpal and proximal phalanx of the fifth finger.

Hand injuries were the focus of Kiely et al's study in 2003. A successive 123 hand injuries were seen in the study period of which forty-one were sustained during hurling matches. [13] Forty of the players were male, with a mean age of 20 years (range 9–53 years). Injury to the dominant hand occurred in 23 cases (56%). Fractures of the bones of the hand accounted for 38 of the injuries (eighteen fractured metacarpals, 14 fractured proximal phalanges and 6 middle or distal phalangeal fractures), with two players suffering dislocations and one player sustaining a laceration of the nail bed. Of the digital fractures, the little finger and the thumb were the most commonly involved. Thirty-three players were managed conservatively, with either neighbour strapping or splinting, and eight players required admission overnight for surgical procedures under general anaesthesia. Two cases had manipulation under anaesthesia, one patient had a nail bed laceration repaired while the remaining five cases necessitated manipulation under anaesthesia plus kirschner wiring [13].

With increased helmet use, hand injuries became the commonest injuries seen in hurlers presenting to hospital. A 2006 study performed in Cork found that in hurlers presenting to the emergency department, the most commonly injured site was the upper extremity distal to the wrist (52.1%) followed by the lower limb (18.4%) and then followed by 27 head injuries (16.6%). [3] A significant number (62%) of the distal upper limb injuries sustained from a blow of a hurley were fractures, compared to soft tissue injury (laceration and ligamentous injury) (n=28/74). The most commonly injured digits were the first (n=16) and the fifth (n=15). Fractures most commonly occurred to the metacarpal bones (n=17, 37%), followed by the proximal phalanges (n=15, 32%), with the middle phalanx the least likely to be fractured (n=4, 8%) and the distal phalanx fractured in only 10 cases (22%) [3].

In a 2006 study of camogie players, self reported injury rates were assessed over a 12 month period of playing and training. Hand injuries were by far the most common type of injury (experienced by 42% of injured players), followed by thigh and shin injuries. Of twenty-two players who suffered a hand injury, only two (9%) were wearing a handguard at the time. One in six players experienced a hand injury over the 12-month period [10].

Muscular and Spinal Injuries

Not all hurling injuries require hospital admission. The majority of these injuries are muscular in nature. In a prospective study of 74 hurlers over one season, the most common type of injury sustained was muscle strain (24.4% of all injuries). [8] The hamstrings were the most common site of strain, accounting for 41%. Other common injuries were contusions (16.3%) and sprains (15.6%) [8].

Spinal injuries, although rare, have also been reported. The most common sport responsible for a spinal injury presenting to an orthopaedic unit was equestrian events (41.8%) followed by rugby (16.3%). Gaelic football (8.1%) and hurling (1.5%) accounted for much smaller numbers [19].

Newly Emerging Injury Patterns

Since the introduction of helmets, new patterns of injury have of course emerged. A 6-month retrospective analysis was carried out of patients attending Cork University Hospital (CUH) with ear lacerations sustained while hurling and identified seven patients. [2] All patients were males with a mean age of 22 years. All wore helmets complying with current legislation including a faceguard and none were using additional ear protection. Injuries in each case were classified as complex, involving lacerations of the anterior skin, cartilage and posterior skin.

Three patients had additional extension of the wound onto the skull in the posterior auricular area. No other injuries were sustained. All patients had their injuries repaired under local anaesthesia in the plastic surgery unit. The potential for the unprotected ear to be injured whilst wearing approved helmets has been newly identified by this study [2].

Player Attitudes to Protective Equipment

Player attitude to protective equipment use has been reported from a number of different studies.

Helmets

When helmets were still optional, a number of factors pertaining to helmet use amongst players were studied by Crowley in 1995. [11] Younger players were significantly more likely to wear helmets with a mean age of 18.7 years for users compared to 20.4 years for non-users. [11] A similar pattern of younger players being more safety-conscious was seen when the helmet wearers were divided on the basis of the use or non-use of a faceguard; the average age of those wearing a faceguard was 17.2 years compared to 19.7 years for those without such protection [11].

When the 45 players from the men's senior intercounty hurling panels of Kilkenny and Waterford were studied, a total of 32 (71%) players wore helmets of which 28 (87.5%) contained faceguards. [9] Of the 28 players with faceguards, 26 (93%) had them added to their original helmet with 5 of these players removing the faceguard at a later date. Two players stated that removal of the faceguard allowed them to hurl better. No player stated that financial cost was a consideration in determining whether to wear a helmet/faceguard. It was notable that almost all players (90.6%) wearing helmets/faceguards had been doing so since playing at underage grades. Ten players (31.3%) stated they began wearing a helmet after sustaining an injury. A single player began wearing a helmet after witnessing an injury [9].

Twenty-three (71.9%) helmet/faceguard wearers felt that wearing a safety apparatus had prevented or at least limited the severity of injuries they had received. [9] Thirty-one (97%) out of 32 players felt the helmet provided them with greater security on the field while 19 (59.4%) players stated that their helmet allowed them to play better. Nineteen (59.4%) also stated that wearing a helmet/faceguard made them take risks during games they would not normally take. When given a choice of safety, comfort and looks as being important factors in helmet design, 25 (78%) stated comfort was a key component of helmet design [9].

Helmet performance was generally rated as good. Twenty-seven (84.4%) players felt that their helmets/faceguards performed well (n = 8) or at least fairly well (n = 19) in warm weather. The figures for wet weather were similar with 90.6% players feeling that they performed well or at least fairly well. Nevertheless 40.6% expressed some sort of frustration with their helmet while 62.5% of players felt they could improve overall helmet design. Nine players admitted discontinuing wear for a prolonged period. Discontinuation was due to discomfort (n = 4), playing badly (n = 2) or interference with vision. Interestingly six players resumed wear after sustaining an injury while a further player resumed his wear after witnessing an injury [9].

The number of camogie players reporting wearing helmets was assessed by Quinn in 2006. [10] Altogether, 74.8% of players reported wearing a helmet all of the time; only 5% never wore a helmet. Direct observation of players in action showed the number observed wearing helmets to be 114/139 (95%), which compared well with the self-reported data. Of those wearing helmets, 96.2% had a faceguard. The most common reason given for not always wearing a helmet was that it was uncomfortable. The great majority (98.6%) of players agreed with the compulsory nature of helmets under the age of 18 [10].

Handguards

In a study of injured hurlers, only 8 (4.9%) regularly used hand protection, while 149 (91.4%) had tried it in the past. [3] Given this high trial-rate with poor uptake, respondents were asked why they had discontinued use of available handguards. Most respondents (n=123, 75.4%) described poor utility citing issues such as bulkiness and diminished dexterity. More than half (n=95, 58.3%) felt that protection was inadequate, offering ineffective hand protection. When asked about the potential interest in new protective equipment, however, 121 (74.2%) felt they would still try a newly designed glove [3].

In Kiely and colleagues hand injury study, thirty-seven of the 41 injured players wore no hand protection, but the four players who used the commercially available glove avoided injury to the specific area protected. [13] The proportion of players wearing the protective device in this series reflected the national trend at the time. Modification of this glove, with reinforcement of the peripheries, may be required to offer better protection for injuries sustained despite wearing the glove.

The number of camogie players who self reported wearing handguards in the Quinn study was also very low at <5%. [10] The numbers directly observed wearing handguards in this study supported this data: only 2.5% (n=3) of players were wearing handguards in the observed matches. The main reasons given for not wearing the handguard were lack of comfort (62.9%), feeling it was unnecessary (40.3%), and feeling it impaired play (5.7%). Despite 42.4% of players reporting having tried wearing a handguard on at least one occasion, 84.9% of players reported never wearing a handguard when playing. This again showed a willingness to try hand protection, but a lack of acceptability of current handguard design [10].

Successful Introduction of Protective Helmets

The early hurling studies had suggested a beneficial role for helmets in reducing head injury rates. [1,12] Work was then undertaken to design suitable protective head protection for hurlers. One of the early researchers into hurling related injury focused on developing handmade helmet proto-types during the period 1979–1983 and then approached the national industrial authority with a proposal to establish an enterprise to produce protective helmets and faceguards for hurlers. [7] This organisation requested reliable epidemiological information regarding the scale and nature of hurling injuries requiring emergency department care. The findings of this study suggested that custom-designed protective headgear was likely to prove most effective in the prevention of hurling injuries while simultaneously being more acceptable to players. [7] In this helmet study, 41% of non-helmeted injured players suffered head injuries compared to just 13% of their helmeted counterparts. Within the helmeted injured players, 21% of those not wearing faceguards suffered head injuries compared to just 3% of those wearing a faceguard. [11] On the basis of data generated from this study, the GAA ruled that the use of full protective headgear was mandatory for all players under 18 years of age from January 2005 onwards. The age limit was then further increased to 21 years from April 2007. [7] This rule required use of helmet and an unmodified faceguard.

The benefits of helmet use were further backed up by subsequent studies. In Murphy's study of facial injuries, the majority of injuries (75%) in the study group occurred when no helmet was worn. [15] The helmet injuries group comprised 25% of injuries. When comparing the helmet with modified faceguards group to helmet with unmodified faceguards group, the results revealed that the modified faceguard group had significantly more injuries. These modified helmets afford less protection as there is less lateral facial coverage and bars are removed to improve vision. This provides insufficient lateral facial coverage and a player using this helmet suffered fractured zygoma and fractured mandible in two successive seasons while wearing this helmet. He required open reduction and internal fixation of both injuries under general anaesthesia [15].

Khan et al, in their study of hurling related eye injuries, compared the data of the 15 months immediately before the GAA's new regulations, rendering it mandatory for all players aged 18 years or under to wear a protective helmet and face mask while playing hurling with the 15 months following this. [4] Of the 43 players injured before 1 January 2005, 12 (27.9%) were aged 18 years or under. Of the 17 players who sustained hurling-related eye injuries between 1 January 2005 and 30 March 2006, only two (11%) were aged 18 years or under. This data represented a significant reduction in the number of hurling-related ocular injuries sustained in players aged 18 years or less following implementation of the new rules [4].

Being aware from the usage survey results of the reluctance of the majority of adult players to use protective headgear, a wall chart was designed to convey the huge increase in the risk of head injury in hurling in the absence of protective equipment. This wall chart was circulated to around 1000 hurling clubs and schools to publicise the importance of protective headgear. [7] The ultimate goal of the programme—a mandatory usage policy for all players—

was eventually achieved during 2008, and it has been enforced since 1 January 2010. On that date, the GAA implemented Rule 4.2 (i) of Part 2 of the Official Guide stating inter alia that "In all Hurling Games and Hurling Practice sessions, it is mandatory for all players to wear a helmet with a facial guard" [7].

As discussed earlier, with the successful implementation of mandatory helmet wearing and a reduction in head injury rates, an unanticipated consequence has been identification of a probable increase in the level of hand injuries, in association with the use of full head protection. [7] This finding may be due to a combination of an increased sense of 'invincibility' due to the substantial risk reduction of head injury (with some players having admitted to taking more risks when playing hurling whilst wearing a helmet [9]) and potentially some degree of temporary visual impedance due to the use of full protective equipment. [7] Consequently, a protective glove was developed and is now available. However, as discussed earlier, there remain some issues with player acceptability of the available hand protection and usage rates are low.

Summary and Conclusion

In summary, hurling is a fast field sport with close player contact. As a result of this, injury is a common occurrence. In keeping with the age range of players playing hurling, those experiencing injury are generally of a young age and injuries can be serious.

Protective equipment was introduced to address the inherent injury risk in hurling. Head injuries were the commonest injury requiring hospital attendance prior to the introduction of helmets. Since 2010 a helmet with full faceguard has been a mandatory requirement for all hurling and camogie players. Head injuries have significantly reduced since the introduction of helmets. The commonest injury now encountered is hand injuries. A protective glove has been developed and introduced on a voluntary basis. Many players have tried this handguard, but few use it consistently citing issues with comfort and usability of the current design. Adaptation of the handguard to address comfort issues and attempt to reduce the risk of hand injury in hurling and camogie remains an issue for the future.

References

[1] Crowley PJ, Condon KC. Analysis of hurling and camogie injuries. *Br. J. Sports Med.,* 1989; 23(3):183.

[2] Martin Smith J, Chan J, Power K et al. Do helmets worn for hurling fail to protect the ear? Identification of an emerging injury pattern. *Br. J. Sports Med.*, 2012; 46(16):1134.

[3] Falvey E, McCrory P, Crowley B et al. Risk factors for hand injury in hurling: a cross-sectional study. 2013, *BMJ Open*; 3(5).

[4] Khan M, Flynn T, O'Connell E et al. The impact of new regulations on the incidence and severity of ocular injury sustained in hurling. *Eye* (Lond), 2008; 22(4):475.

[5] Maclean. A survey of shinty injuries in the Highlands during 1987-1988. *Br. J. Sports Med.,* 1989; 23(3):179.

[6] King S. The clash of the ash in Foreign fields: hurling abroad. Shannon, Co. Clare: *Seamus J.* King, 1998.

[7] Crowley PJ, Crowley MJ. Dramatic impact of using protective equipment on the level of hurling-related head injuries: an ultimately successful 27-year programme. *Br. J. Sports Med.*, 2014; 48(2): 147.

[8] Watson A. Sports injuries in the game of hurling. A one-year prospective study. *Am. J. Sports Med.*, 1996; 24(3):323.

[9] Hennessy B, Murray I, O'Connor K et al. Prevailing attitude amongst current senior intercounty hurlers to head and facial protection: a pilot study. *Ir. J. med. Sci.*, 2007; 176(4):279.

[10] Quinn EM, Bradley CP. Injury prevention in camogie: Current trends in the use of protective equipment. *Eur. J. Sport Sci.,* 2012;12:185.

[11] Crowley PJ, Crowley MJ, Dardouri H, Condon KC. Value of wearing head protection gear while playing hurling. *Br. J. Sports Med.*, 1995; 29(3): 191.

[12] Cuddihy B, Hurley M. Contact sports and injury. *Ir. Med. J.*, 1990; 83(3):98.

[13] 13, Kiely PD, Ashraff M, O'Grady P et al. Hurling-related hand injuries. Injury, 2003; 34(8):561.

[14] O'Connor K, Hennessy B, Murray I et al. Prevalence of head and facial trauma in current senior intercounty hurlers. *Ir. Med. J.,* 2006; 99(1):17.

[15] Murphy C, Ahmed I, Mullarkey C, Kearns G. Maxillofacial and dental injuries sustained in hurling. *Ir. Med. J.,* 2010; 103(6):174.

[16] Flynn TH, Fennessy K, Horgan N et al. Ocular injury in hurling. *Br. J. Sports Med.,* 2005; 39(8):493.

[17] Lynch P, Rowan. Eye injury and sport: sport-related eye injuries presenting to an eye casualty department throughout 1995. *Ir. Med. J.*, 1997; 90(3):112.

[18] Walker T, Byrne S, Donnellan J et al. West of Ireland facial injury study. Part 2. *Br. J.* Oral Maxillofac Surg, 2012; 50(7):e99.

[19] Boran S, Lenehan B, Street J at al. A 10-year review of sports-related spinal injuries. Ir. J. med. Sci., 2011; 180(4):859.

[20] Delaney R, Falvey E, Kalimuthu S et al. Orthopaedic admissions due to sports and recreation injuries. *Ir. Med. J.,* 2009; 102(2):40.

[21] Carroll S, Jawad S, West M, O'Connor T. One hundred and ten sports related facial fractures. *Br. J. Sports Med.*, 1995; 29(3): 194.

[22] Gaelic Athletic Association. Official guide - Part 2. Containing Playing Rules of Hurling and Football, revised and corrected up to date, and published by authority of the Central Council. 2012. Central Council of the Association, Dublin, Ireland. http://www.gaa.ie/content/documents/publications/official_guides/Official_Guide_2012_Part2.pdf [accessed 24th August 2014].

In: Sports Injuries
Editor: Gabrielle Hopkins

ISBN: 978-1-63463-305-5

Chapter 6

RESISTANCE TRAINING'S ROLE IN THE PREVENTION OF SPORTS INJURIES

Ina Shaw, Ph.D. and Brandon S. Shaw, Ph.D.
University of Johannesburg, Johannesburg, South Africa

ABSTRACT

It is generally accepted that regular scientifically-designed resistance training programs result in numerous benefits in both competitive and recreational athletes including improvements in muscle strength and power, increases in muscle size all leading to improvements in sports performance. In addition, resistance training has also been suggested to reduce the risk for musculoskeletal injuries or even reduce the severity of such injuries in athletes. In this regard, resistance training can strengthen muscles, bones and connective tissue making them less susceptible to damage and more able to withstand the demands of sport and physical activity. Although studies reporting the direct effect of resistance training on injury rate reduction are limited, the physiological adaptations seen consequent to resistance training on muscles, bones and connective tissue does imply enhanced protection against musculoskeletal injuries. Reducing the incidence of injury by engaging in a resistance training program is as beneficial for the non-competitive beginner as it is for the competitive athlete. Thankfully, many competitive and recreational athletes already perform resistance training as a part of their usual conditioning programs. However, there is an increasing need to engage in resistance exercises that reproduce the performance of the sport and/or motion specific activities. These specific types of resistance exercises should also be performed following the testing of athletes for agonist and antagonist muscle strength imbalances as such data can be utilized to identify athletes with a predisposition for injury. In these cases, resistance training may then be performed to correct the observed imbalance and hopefully reduce the incidence and/or severity of future injury. While evidence suggests that a targeted resistance-based approach can prevent musculoskeletal injuries or even reduce the severity, recent evidence suggests that resistance can also be utilized to accelerate recovery from such injuries and is increasingly being used in this role as an excellent alternative method of rehabilitating sports injuries. However, it must be noted that the improper execution of resistance exercises can themselves be cause for injury, especially in the youth. As such, resistance-focused workouts should be performed with proper form and technique or under the supervision of qualified and certified trainers. In conclusion, despite the old belief of resistance training being ineffective and unsafe, resistance training has been shown to decrease sport injuries and their severity, rehabilitation time relative to non-resistance trained individuals and should be considered as an important component to include in any fitness or sport-performance program, even in the youth due to their ever-lengthening and increasingly earlier competitive careers.

Keywords: Safety, strength training, weight training

INTRODUCTION

The benefits of resistance training in both competitive and recreational athletes have been well documented over the past 20 years. Resistance training is commonly referred to as weight training or incorrectly as strength training. Improvements in muscle strength and power, increase in muscle size, and improvement in sports performance are common benefits resulting from resistance training programs. In addition, resistance training has also been suggested in the promotion of general health, the reduction of the risk of developing chronic diseases, such as dyslipidemia, and even in their rehabilitation (Shaw, Shaw & Goon, 2011). While resistance training is more commonly associated with injury rehabilitation, resistance training is increasingly becoming more important in the prevention of musculoskeletal injuries, or perhaps contributes to the reduction of severity of such injuries (Hoffman, n.d).

Resistance training is the use of resistance to muscular contraction to build the strength, anaerobic endurance and size of skeletal muscles. Resistance training can take the guise of strength training, power training (either multiple effort or single effort), hypertrophy training or muscular endurance training (Baechle, Earle & Wathen, 2008), each resulting in their own adaptations to the musculoskeletal system which may reduce the risk for musculoskeletal injuries or even reduce the severity of such injuries in athletes (Table 1).

Table 1. Resistance training load, repetitions, sets and rest periods for resistance training program design based on the training goals

Training Goal	Load (%1-RM)	Repetitions	Sets	Rest period length
Strength	≥ 85	≤ 6	2-6	2-5 minutes
Power (single effort)	80-90 (at maximum speed)	1-2	3-5	2-5 minutes
Power (multiple effort)	75-85 (at maximum speed)	3-5	3-5	2-5 minutes
Hypertrophy	67-85	6-12	3-6	30 seconds to 1.5 minutes
Muscular endurance	≤ 67	≥ 12	2-3	30 seconds or less

Adapted from Baechle, Earle & Wathen, 2008.

Musculoskeletal Benefits of Resistance Training in the Prevention of Sports Injuries

Luckily, many competitive and recreational athletes already perform resistance training as a part of their conditioning programs in an attempt to improve their sport performance. These conditioning programs utilizing resistance training aim to increase muscular strength and hypertrophy which may also aid in the prevention of injuries. This is so since research indicates that resistance training promotes growth and/or increases in the strength of ligaments, tendons, tendon to bone and ligament to bone junction strength, joint cartilage, the connective tissue sheaths within muscle and causes an increase in bone mineral content and therefore may aid in injury prevention (Fleck & Falkel, 1986). This protective effect of resistance training on musculoskeletal properties may reduce the risk of developing both chronic/overuse and acute injuries (Bahr et al., 2012; Fleck & Falkel, 1986).

Although studies reporting the direct effect of resistance training on injury rate reduction are limited, the physiological adaptations on muscle, bone and connective tissue observed following resistance training imply an enhanced protection against injury for individuals who participate in such a resistance training program (Hoffman, n.d).

Muscular Adaptations Following Resistance Training in the Prevention of Sports Injuries

Resistance training has an important role in reducing the risk for musculoskeletal injuries and does so via several effects on skeletal muscle. Most importantly, resistance training, and specifically strength and power training, results in less muscle fibres being used at a given submaximal load (Ploutz et al., 1994) and thus fewer fibres are susceptible to injury. Further, these increases in strength reduce injuries in that an increase in muscular strength results in an increase in functional and sport-specific ability. This increase in functional and sport-specific ability results in a decrease in risk for sports injuries in that these abilities can only be maintained if there is sufficient muscle strength to compensate for any decreases in accuracy of modulation and activation of muscles (Van Der Esch et al., 2007). This type of resistance training also results in a higher maximal effort and rate of force development (Oliveira et al., 2013), which results in a higher tolerance to external and internal forces.

Resistance training, mainly in the form of hypertrophy training, also causes significant increases in muscle hypertrophy, which refers to the growth and increase of the size of muscle cells. These increases in muscle hypertrophy may then assist in the reduction of sports injuries in that hypertrophied muscles are better able to support metabolism and healing from normal, minor breakdown during exercise and even assist in the speed and quality of recovery from sports injuries. In addition, the increased soft tissue mass associated with hypertrophied muscle are better able to absorb impact during direct trauma (Donahue, 2001), such as a tackle or a blow from a ball or stick. Conditioned muscles' intensities and peak timings during activities also become more coordinated to absorb landing impact during running or jumping (Iida et al., 2011), effectively reducing the risk of developing injuries during these activities.

Resistance training also has an important role in reducing the risk for musculoskeletal injuries related to muscle imbalance. This imbalance can either be in the form of an agonist to antagonist ratio (i.e., elbow flexors/elbow extensors) or a bilateral comparison (i.e., right and left elbow flexors). As such, the correction of an existing imbalance through a targeted resistance training program is important in reducing an individual's risk for developing a sports injury (Hoffman, n.d).

Connective Tissue Adaptations Following Resistance Training in the Prevention of Sports Injuries

Connective tissue connects, supports, binds, or separates other tissues or organs and these tissues typically have relatively few cells embedded in an amorphous matrix, often with collagen or other fibers. It is essential for any athlete or health professional to note that muscle strength is limited by the ability of the tendon to handle the force generated by the muscle and that the muscular system is affected by the strength of the ligaments to stabilize the joints involved in any movement (Bahr et al., 2012), hence a systematic and long-term injury prevention program should be in place for all athletes in order to optimize performance and lengthen an athlete's competitive career.

To date, there has been little research conducted on the direct effect of resistance training on connective tissue adaptations (Hoffman, n.d; Stone, 1988). However, those that have completed such studies have demonstrated that 1) physical activity can increase connective tissue strength and mass, 2) activation of the antigravity muscles must be accomplished to adequately stimulate connective tissue, and 3) the volume, intensity, and load-bearing nature of the exercise training are important factors in causing connective tissue adaptations (Stone, 1988). These increases in the size of connective tissues are thought to be the result of an increase in the collagen content within the connective tissue sheaths. Interestingly, although collagen content increases with training, increases in collagen content are proportional to the increase in muscle, hence the need for hypertrophy resistance training in any injury prevention program (Hoffman, n.d).

Bone Adaptations Following Resistance Training in the Prevention of Sports Injuries

The main function of bone is to provide the mechanical integrity for locomotion and protection while bone mass and architecture are adjusted to control the strains produced by mechanical load and muscular activity. As such, a low bone mass results in increased risk of fractures. Bone is living tissue and it has the ability to remodel and adapt to the physical stresses imposed on it (Hoffman, n.d) and allows the bones to become more capable of taking on an increased load before becoming injured. In addition, following an injury, the associated bone loss may be lessened dependant on the type and severity of the injury. Further, bone loss associated with an injury is dependent on the existing level of bone mass prior to injury and as such, a higher bone mass may not only reduce the severity of an injury, but facilitate a more rapid return to sport.

Although bone mass and architecture will respond to many types of training programs, especially those with high strain such as jumping or running, it does appear that resistance training provides the greatest osteogenic (increase in bone mineral density) effect (Carter & Hinton, 2014; Suominen, 2006). This increased bone mass then effectively reduces the risk of developing osteoporosis, fractures or other conditions related to bone deterioration commonly seen in athletes due to their training or nutritional regimes or when bone tissue critical levels are exceeded during training and competition. In response to loading of the bone, whether created by muscular contractions or other methods of mechanical forces, the bone begins a process of bone modelling which involves the manufacture of protein molecules that are deposited in the spaces between bone cells. This leads to the creation of a bone matrix which ultimately becomes mineralized as calcium phosphate crystals, resulting in the bone acquiring its rigid structure. This new bone formation occurs chiefly on the outer surface of the bone, or periosteum (Kravitz, n.d.).

However, as with any type of exercise, these adaptations are site-specific (Suominen, 2006) resulting in a need for an appropriate needs analysis and concomitant, evidence-based resistance training program design. In this regard, resistance training for muscular strength appears to be positively related to bone mineral content and bone strength. Thus, muscular strength improves bone strength as well. However, it is not clear whether the relative improvements in bone and muscle strength during a resistance training program are similar (Hoffman, n.d). When designing injury-prevention programs to increase bone growth, programs must incorporate resistance training in the form of strength training. These resistance training exercises should be structural in nature such as squats and lunges, which direct the forces through the axial skeleton and allow greater loads to be utilized (Conroy & Earle, 1994). In this regard, the critical magnitude or intensity (minimal essential strain) required to produce an effective stimulus for bone remodelling appears to be a 1 repetition maximum (RM) to 10 RM load (Kraemer, 1994).

Neural Adaptations Following Resistance Training in the Prevention of Sports Injuries

Although the effect of resistance training on muscle morphology has been thoroughly examined, less is known about the specific neural mechanisms responsible for training-induced increases in the nervous system (Del Balso & Cafarelli, 2007). However, it is known that resistance training may produce adaptations in the neuromuscular chain from the individual muscle fibres through to the higher brain centres (Ratamess, 2014). These adaptations are critical to injury prevention in that an increase in neural drive is essential for maximal strength and power which itself is needed to optimally overcome internal and external forces which could cause an injury. Increases in neural drive are thought to occur in response to increases in agonist muscle recruitment, increases in firing rate, improved timing and discharge of high-intensity muscular contractions, and a reduction in inhibitory neuromuscular mechanisms (Ratamess, 2014).

While increases in muscular strength among initially untrained subjects are relatively easily attained taking place during the earlier weeks of strength training mainly due to neural adaptations, there is a gradually increasing contribution of hypertrophic factors as the training proceeds (Häkkinen, 1989). Thus, there is a need for any injury-prevention program to include resistance training that focuses on both strength and hypertrophy training. In addition, resistance training in the form of power training should also be included in any injury-prevention program since it has been found that explosive training is able to produce improvements in explosive force associated with increased rapid activation of trained muscles, in addition to a more economical sport-specific performance (Mikkola et al., 2007), both of which may contribute to a reduced risk for musculoskeletal injuries or even reduce the severity of injuries in athletes.

Targeted Resistance Training for the Prevention of Sport Injuries

There are many different issues when designing injury-prevention programs. It is believed that it is important first to recognise the injury pattern characteristics of the sport before it is possible to design a targeted resistance program for the prevention of sport injuries (Parkkari, Kujala & Kannus, 2001).

While resistance training programs must include the major muscles and muscle groups required for a particular sport in order to reduce the risk for musculoskeletal injuries or even reduce the severity of such injuries, resistance training programs must also include all synergist, stabilizer and antagonist muscles (Fleck & Falkel, 1986). This will ensure that all muscles involved in a sport or a particular movement in that sport is enhanced. In addition, each particular sport requires a specific expression of movement i.e., strength, power (either multiple effort or single effort), muscular endurance training or more likely, a combination of movements. In this regard, endurance sports, like middle distance running, require specific muscles (such as the lower extremity) to perform under strain for longer periods and patterns of movement. This specificity of movement in each sport dictates that a needs analysis be performed to determine the requirements and characteristics of the sport and the individual player prior to engaging in a resistance training program to improve performance and to reduce the risk of injury from that particular sport (Baechle, Earle & Wathen, 2008). Such screening of an athlete can be utilized to identify athletes possessing a predisposition for injury. Only then can resistance training be performed to correct the imbalance and therefore reduce the incidence of injury (Fleck & Falkel, 1986).

Risks Associated with Resistance Training

Although regular exercise helps reduce the risk for musculoskeletal injuries or even reduce the severity of injuries, musculoskeletal complications increase transiently during strenuous physical activity compared with the risk at other times (Thompson et al., 2007). The risks associated with resistance training have caused many individuals and athletes to avoid resistance training. However, resistance training, as with lifting any heavy object or engaging in any exercise, comes with its dangers. In this regard, somewhat paradoxically, while resistance training can prevent or reduce the severity of injuries, common injuries from resistance training include musculoskeletal injuries ranging from muscle soreness to muscle and/or tendon strains, ligament sprains and bone fractures (Almeida et al., 1999). However, numerous injuries occur from individuals dropping weights on themselves. Irrespective of the type of injury, resistance training-related injuries are preventable and being aware of the possible dangers of resistance training may assist in the prevention of such injuries. A common cause of musculoskeletal injuries sustained during resistance training pertains to excessively overloading muscles, either by lifting excessively heavy weight or training the same muscle or muscle group too frequently. This is especially common in beginners.

Resistance training is commonly considered inappropriate for cardiovascular health due to high-intensity resistance training displaying a linear relationship with blood pressure in that the higher the intensity of the resistance training, the greater the elevation in blood pressure and associated cardiovascular health risks. This makes high-intensity resistance training particularly unsuitable for individuals who are hypertensive. Further, significant increases in blood pressure during all forms of exercise should be avoided if at all possible. However, low- or moderate-intensity resistance training offers a solution in that it enables hypertensive patients to reap the benefits of resistance training without experiencing dangerous increases in blood pressure (Shaw & Shaw, 2006). A less commonly known risk of high-intensity resistance training is aortic dissection, in which the wall of the aorta tears, allowing blood to flow between the layers of the wall of the aorta and ultimately forcing the layers apart. Aortic dissection, which is a risk for anyone who does resistance training, is directly related to the degree of physical exertion. High-intensity exercise, particularly heavy resistance training, dramatically increases the risks of aortic dissection.

The risks associated with high-intensity resistance training are well known and documented. These risks have created a serious conflict for fitness professionals because individuals need the associated benefits of muscle development, but for some the risks may simply outweigh the benefits. As a result, many trainers simply avoid resistance training with their high-risk clients and/or modify resistance training programs to the point of being overly cautious. However, low- or moderate-intensity resistance training performed using specific guidelines offers a safe and plausible way to provide all recreational and professional athletes, regardless of risk factors, the benefits of resistance training. This is so since, as with any form of exercise, resistance training can take the guise of low- moderate- or high-intensity training, all of which offer their own unique benefits to injury prevention.

Resistance Training in Young Athletes in the Prevention of Sports Injuries

Although resistance training was once considered inappropriate for youth, there is an increasing body of evidence which demonstrates the safety and efficacy of such training for children and adolescents, provided that the training program is well designed and supervised by qualified professionals.

Previously, resistance training has been restricted in children and adolescents due to possible deleterious effects on the physis, or growth plate. These concerns about the effects of resistance training arise since the physis is relatively weaker than the surrounding bone and it has been speculated that resistance training places children and adolescents with immature skeletons at risk for growth plate injury from forces that would not harm an adult. However, although the avoidance of resistance training by children and adolescents is theoretically appealing, empirical data indicates that well-designed and properly supervised resistance training programs are not associated with increased risk of acute injury and preseason conditioning programs which include resistance training have even been found to reduce sports-related injuries in young athletes (Milone et al., 2013). In addition, it is imperative to include resistance training in a child or adolescent's exercise program not only for overall health but also conditioning and competitiveness. This is so since the benefits of resistance training for an injury-prevention program in children and adolescents include, increases in strength gains, which increases joint stability, improved motor performance, which enhances not only performance but increases proprioceptive ability, stability, and efficiency of movement and early exposure to well-designed and supervised resistance training provides exposure to appropriate and correct coaching techniques, that may be useful in adult life.

In the past and in most cases, low- to moderate- intensities are usually recommended for children and adolescents when engaging in resistance training. However, evidence is increasingly demonstrating that strength training is a relatively safe and healthy practice for children and adolescents, provided that they observe the same safety rules (i.e., medical clearance, proper instruction from a qualified professional and progressive overload) as that of their adult counterparts (Barbieri & Zaccagni, 2013). In addition, several studies provide consistent findings of improved motor skills and body composition, in terms of increased fat free mass, reduced fat mass and enhanced bone health in children and adolescents following resistance training (Barbieri & Zaccagni, 2013), all of which can contribute to a child' or adolescent's athletic performance and competitiveness.

Poor Compliance Associated with Resistance-Based Injury-Prevention Programs

When designing any injury-prevention program, irrespective of the mode of exercise, a chief consideration is that compliance is difficult to achieve. In this regard, several studies demonstrating the ineffectiveness of injury-prevention programs are thought to be a result of poor compliance with the prevention programme among athletes. This means that major efforts are required by coaches, strength and conditioning specialists and health professionals in order to motivate athletes to engage in such programs. A possible explanation for poor compliance, especially for resistance-based injury prevention programs, may be based on the finding that individuals more readily adhere to an exercise program when that program is deemed enjoyable (Heyward, 1997) and many individuals may prefer aerobic-type exercise as opposed to resistance training. As such, it is essential when designing injury-prevention programs to consider and convey the simultaneous potential of such programs in enhancing athletic performance.

Conclusion

Although many epidemiological studies on the role of resistance training in the prevention of sports injuries display methodological problems that make conclusions questionable (Feiring & Derscheid, 1989), evidence exists that conditioning programs, especially those in the preseason, should include resistance training irrespective of the sport or the age of the athlete in an attempt to improve the structural integrity of the joint as well as the musclulotendinous unit. Reducing the incidence or the severity of injuries by engaging in a resistance training program is as beneficial for the non-competitive athlete as it is for the professional athlete. However, attention should be given to the target populations and the specificity of the programs related to the requirements of the sport and the strengths and weaknesses of the individual athlete. This is because a more specific and adequate muscle function is thought to help in the prevention of injuries (Feiring & Derscheid, 1989). As such, athletes and health professionals should understand the issues that need to be taken into account for appropriate resistance training programme design.

REFERENCES

Almeida, S.A., Trone, D.W., Leone, D.M., Shaffer, R.A., Patheal, S.L. & Long, K. (1999). Gender differences in musculoskeletal injury rates: a function of symptom reporting? *Medicine and Science in Sports and Exercise,* 31(12), 1807-1812.

Baechle, T.R., Earle, R.W. & Wathen, D. (2008). Resistance training. In: Baechle, T.R. & Earle, R.W. (Eds.). *Essentials of strength training and conditioning* (3rd ed.). Champaign, IL: Human Kinetics.

Bahr, R., Blair, S., Cook, J., Crossley, K., McConnell, J., McCrory, P. & Noakes, T.K. (2012). *Brukner & Khan's clinical sports medicine* (4th ed.). Australia: McGraw-Hill.

Barbieri, D. & Zaccagni, L. (2013). Strength training for children and adolescents: benefits and risks. *Collegium Antropologicum*, 37(Suppl 2), 219-225.

Carter, M.I. & Hinton, P.S. (2014). Physical activity and bone health, *Missouri Medicine*, 111(1), 59-64.

Conroy, B. P., & Earle, R. W. (1994). Bone, muscle and connective tissue adaptations to physical activity. In: Baechle, T.R. & Earle, R.W. (Eds.). *Essentials of strength training*Champaign, IL: Human Kinetics.

Del Balso, C. & Cafarelli, E. (2007). Adaptations in the activation of human skeletal muscle induced by short-term isometric resistance training. *Journal of Applied Physiology*, 103(1), 402-411.

Donahue, S.W. (2001). The role of muscular force and fatigue in stress fractures. In: Burr, D.B. & Milgrom, C. (Eds.). *Musculoskeletal fatigue and stress fractures*. Lewis Publishers: Boca Raton.

Feiring, D.C. & Derscheid, G.L. (1989). The role of preseason conditioning in preventing athletic injuries. *Clinics in Sports Medicine*, 8(3), 361-372.

Fleck, S.J. & Falkel, J.E. (1986). Value of resistance training for the reduction of sports injuries. *Sports Medicine*, 3(1), 61-68.

Häkkinen, K. (1989). Neuromuscular and hormonal adaptations during strength and power training. A review. *Journal of Sports Medicine and Physical Fitness*, 29(1), 9-26.

Heyward, V.H. (1997). *Advanced fitness assessment and exercise prescription.* Champaign, IL: Human Kinetics.

Hoffman, J. (n.d). *ACSM current comment: Resistance training and injury prevention.* Accessed: http://www.acsm.org/docs/current-comments/rtandip.pdf. 5 July 2014.

Iida, Y., Kanehisa, H., Inaba, Y. & Nakazawa, K. (2011). Activity modulations of trunk and lower limb muscles during impact-absorbing landing. *Journal of Electromyography and Kinesiology*, 21(4), 602-609.

Kraemer, W. J. (1994). General adaptations to resistance and endurance training programs. In: Baechle, T.R. & Earle, R.W. (Eds.). *Essentials of strength training*Champaign, IL: Human Kinetics.

Kravitz, L. (n.d.). *Resistance training: Adaptations and health implications.* Accessed: http://www.unm.edu/~lkravitz/Article%20folder/resistben.html. 20 Junc 2014.

Mikkola, J.S., Rusko, H.K., Nummela, A.T., Paavolainen, L.M. & Hakkinen, K. (2007). Concurrent endurance and explosive type strength training increases activation and fast force production of leg extensor muscles in endurance athletes. *Journal of Strength and Conditioning Research*, 21(2), 613-620.

Milone, M.T., Bernstein, J., Freedman, K.B. & Tjoumakaris, F. (2013). There is no need to avoid resistance training (weight lifting) until physeal closure. *Physician and Sports Medicine*, 41(4), 101-105.

Moro, T., Bianco, A., Faigenbaum, A.D. & Paoli, A. (2014). Pediatric resistance training: current issues and concerns. *Minerva Pediatrica*, 66(3), 217-227.

Oliveira F.B.D., Oliveira, A.S.C., Rizatto, G.F. & Denadai, B.S. (2013). Resistance training for explosive and maximal strength: Effects on early and late rate of force development. *Journal of Sports Science and Medicine*, 12, 402-408.

Parkkari, J., Kujala, U.M. & Kannus P. (2001). Is it possible to prevent sports injuries?: Review of controlled clinical trials and recommendations for future work. *Sports Medicine*, 31, 985-995.

Ploutz , L L., Tesch , P.A., Biro, R. L. & Dudley, G.A. (1994). Effect of resistance training on muscle use during exercise. *Journal of Applied Physiology*, 76, 1675-1681.

Ratamess, N.A. (2014). Adaptations to anaerobic training programs. In: Baechle, T.R. & Earle, R.W. (Eds.). *Essentials of strength training*Champaign, IL: Human Kinetics.

Shaw, B.S., Shaw, I. & Goon, D.T. (2011). Resistance training and blood lipid regulation: A review of the evidence. *Medicina Dello Sport*, 64(4), 511-521.

Shaw, I. & Shaw, B.S. (2006). Effects of Aerobic, Resistance and Combination Exercise Training on Resting Blood Pressure: A Comparative Study. *African Journal for Physical, Health Education, Recreation and Dance*, 12(4), 384-393.

Stone, M.H. (1988). Implications for connective tissue and bone alterations resulting from resistance exercise training. *Medicine and Science in Sports and Exercise*, 20(5 Suppl), S162-S168.

Suominen, H. (2006). Muscle training for bone strength. *Aging Clinic and Experimental Research*, 18(2), 85-93.

Ter Stege, M.H., Dallinga, J.M., Benjaminse, A. & Lemmink, K.A. (2014). Effect of interventions on potential, modifiable risk factors for knee injury in team ball sports: A systematic review. *Sports Medicine*, Accessed http://link.springer.com/article/10.1007%2 Fs40279-014-0216-4. 05 July 2014.

Thompson, P.D., Franklin, B.A., Balady, G.J., Blair, S.N., Corrado, D. Estes, N.A. 3rd, Fulton, J.E., Gordon, N.F., Haskell, W.L., Link, M.S., Maron, B.J., Mittleman, M.A., Pelliccia, A., Wenger, N.K., Willich, S.N., Costa, F., American Heart Association Council on Nutrition, Physical Activity, and Metabolism; American Heart Association Council on Clinical Cardiology & American College of Sports Medicine. (2007). Exercise and acute cardiovascular events placing the risks into perspective: A scientific statement from the American Heart Association Council on Nutrition, Physical Activity, and Metabolism and the Council on Clinical Cardiology. *Circulation*, 115(17), 2358-2368.

Van Der Esch, M., Steultjens, M., Harlaar, J., Knol, D., Lems, W. & Dekker, J. (2007). Joint proprioception, muscle strength, and functional ability in patients with osteoarthritis of the knee. *Arthritis & Rheumatism (Arthritis Care & Research)*, 57(5), 787-793.

Reviewed by: Prof G.A. Brown

In: Sports Injuries
Editor: Gabrielle Hopkins
ISBN: 978-1-63463-305-5

Chapter 7

Intrinsic Risk Factors That Predispose the Knee Joint to Injury

Terry Jeremy Ellapen, Ph.D.
University of Kwa Zulu-Natal, Westville Campus,
Faculty of Health Science, Department of Biokinetics
and Exercise Science, South Africa

Abstract

The objective of this chapter is to enlighten developing sport medicine practitioners and students on the impact of various intrinsic risk factors that can predispose an athlete to knee pain and injury. Athletes are subjected to both extrinsic (external) and intrinsic (internal) factors that facilitate injury. The pathomechanics of intrinsic factors is not investigated frequently by the sporting fraternity. This chapter reviews the following intrinsic risk factors of knee injury: tibio-femoral alignment in both the sagittal and frontal planes, patella-femoral orientation within the femoral trochlear and the presence of deviant quadriceps, A-angle and torsion angles. The non-invasive clinical techniques that can be used to determine risk of injury and possible soft tissue that has been damaged, will be described. Kendall protocol for lower limb alignment in both the frontal and sagittal planes is used to determine the presence of genu varum (bow leg), genu valgum (knock knees) and genu recurvatum (hyper-extension of the tibio-femoral joint). The presence of the abovementioned clinical conditions is also related to the asymmetrical strength of the surrounding musculature and flaccid ligaments. Prentice's patella orientation techniques are used to identify abnormal patella orientation within femoral trochlear, such as patella alta, baja and medial squinting. The Livingstone and Spaulding technique was used to measure quadriceps angle, while the author uses Prentice's technique to measure the A-angle. Techniques to measure torsion angles are also included.

INTRODUCTION

Consistent physical activity and sport participation is essential for physiological health and mental wellbeing. Regular physical activity reduces the risk of hypokinetic diseases such as diabetes mellitus, coronary heart disease, osteoporosis and lower back pain. [1] Unfortunately, however, participation in sport and physical activity lends itself to injuries, although it must be stressed that the benefits outweigh the associated maladies. [1,2] There are many risk factors that predispose the sport enthusiast to injury, and these are classified as either extrinsic or intrinsic. Intrinsic risk factors are person-dependent factors (body mass, skeletal alignment, muscle strength) and rarely cause injuries, but significantly increase the risk of injury. [1] Extrinsic factors include environmental conditions (extreme heat and/or cold, running or playing surface) and sport equipment that predispose people to injury. This chapter will predominantly deal with the intrinsic risk factors that predispose the knee joint to injury, misalignment of the lower limb and patellar orientation.

A basic comprehension of anatomy and kinesiology is required to appreciate how intrinsic risk factors adversely influence the health of the knee joint. This joint forms the connection between the femur (thigh), the tibia and patella (knee cap). It consists of two joints; the tibio-femoral and patella-femoral joints. Where the tibia and femur meet constitutes the tibio-femoral joint, which is not a true hinge joint, with, the medial condyle of the femur being more developed than the lateral condyle. [3,4] This variation in condylar mass allows the tibia to externally rotate onto the femur during open kinetic chain knee extension, often referred to as the screw home mechanism. [4] The alignment of the tibio-femoral joint influences the kinesiology of the patella-femoral joint, with the patella articulating within the trochlear of the femur during knee flexion and extension.

Various ligaments connect the tibia to the femur, with the main ligaments being the anterior cruciate (ACL), posterior cruciate (PCL), medial collateral

(MCL) and lateral collateral (LCL). Table 1 indicates the functions of these ligaments.

Table 1. Functions of the main ligaments

Ligament	Function
Anterior cruciate (ACL)	• resist anterior translation of the tibia relative to a fixed femur (open kinetic chain exercise), • posterior translation of the femur relative to a fixed tibia (closed kinetic chain exercise), • act as a secondary valgus and varus stabilizer to the MCL and LCL respectively [4]
Posterior cruciate (PCL)	• resistance to posterior translation of tibia relative to a fixed femur, • anterior translation of the femur to a fixed femur [4]
Medial collateral (MCL)	• resists valgus stress, • excessive external rotation of the tibia on the femur
Lateral collateral (LCL)	• resists varus stress, • excessive internal rotation of the tibia on femur [4]

The quadriceps femoris extends the tibio-femoral joint, while the hamstrings flex the tibio-femoral joint. The quadriceps femoris comprises of the vastus medialis, vastus lateralis, intermediate vastus and rectus femoris. [5] The hamstrings muscle constituents are biceps femoris, semimembranosus and semitendinosus. The abductors and adductors act as synergists to knee flexion and extension. The adductor muscles consist of the gracilis, adductor brevis, adductor magnus, adductor longus and pectineus, while the abductor muscles consist of the tensor fascia latae and the gluteus maximus. [5]

Identifying the intrinsic risk factors that can predispose people to injuries include:

i. Lower limb postural analyses,
ii. Abnormal force couples of musculature around the knee joint,
iii. Special non-invasive clinical tests.

1. Lower Limb Postural Analyses

The lower limb analyses involve frontal and sagittal plane assessments according to the protocol of Kendall et al., with the frontal plane assessment including anterior and posterior views. [6] The anterior frontal plane analysis indicates the presence of genu valgum or varum.

Genu valgum is the frontal plane angle that is formed between the femur and tibia during knee extension, and normally ranges between 170-175°. [4,7] Excessive genu valgum is known as knock knees, and is an appearance of tibial deviation away from the midline. [4] Genu valgum increases the ligament laxity of the MCL and ACL, and the compression of the lateral meniscus. [4,5,8,9,10] The ACL and MCL laxity can be assessed by the anterior drawer's test and the valgus stress test, respectively. [11] Meniscal compression injury can be determined by the McMurry meniscal compression test. [11,12]

Genu varum is an abnormal frontal plane angle formed between the femur and the lateral aspect of the tibia, and is known as bow leggedness, with an angle greater than 180°. Genu varum increases the laxity of the LCL and medial meniscus compression. [5] LCL laxity can be assessed using the varus stress test. [11] Sagittal plane observation identifies the presence of genu recurvatum (marked hyperextension of the knee). [6] Genu recurvatum increases the laxity of the ACL predisposing ligament sprains, and, is usually identified by the postural analyses. [6]

Due to the predisposition of genu valgum and/or varum, the femoral muscles' symmetrical force couple relationship becomes altered. [8]

Observing the patella position within the trochlea involves identifying patella normal, alta and/or baja. [8] In the normal patellae, the patella lies within the femoral trochlear. The ratio of the patella's height to patellar tendon length is equal. Patella alta occurs when the patella lies superior to the femoral trochlear, whilst patella baja is the inferior lying patella. [7,8] When the patella does not track within the trochlea patellofemoral pain is produced. [4] In patella alta, the ratio of the height of the patella to the patellar tendon's length exceeds the normal 1:1 ratio. [8]

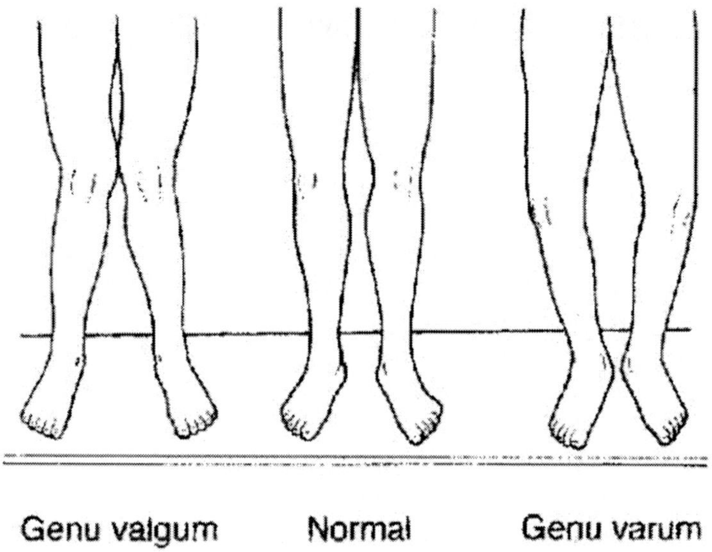

Figure 1. Visual illustration of genu valgum, normal and genu varum tibia femoral alignment (www.google.co.za/url?).

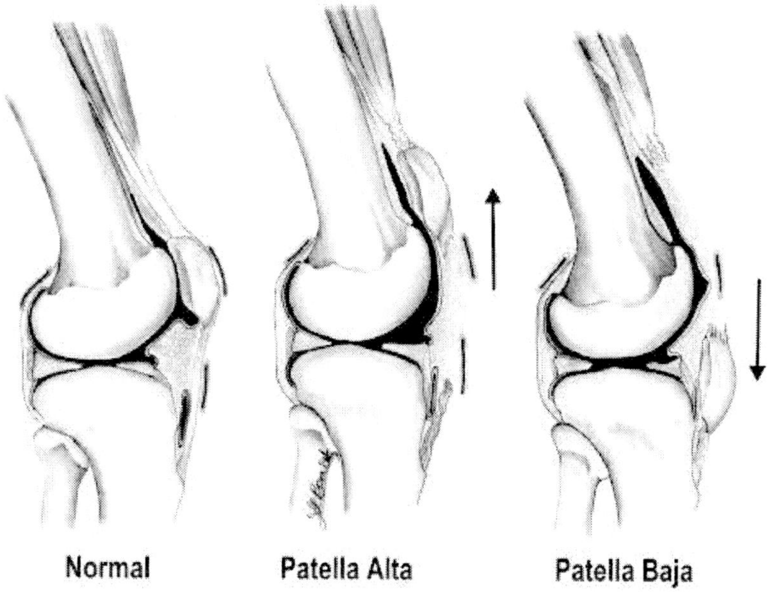

Figure 2. Visual illustration of patella positions (normal, patella baja and patella alta) (www.google.co.za/url?).

2. Abnormal Force Couples of Musculature Around the Knee Joint

Abnormal force couples of the musculature around the knee joint relate to their asymmetrical length tension relationships. This abnormal resting length tension of the musculature initiates patellofemoral pain. [13,14,15] The tensor fascia latae, vastus lateralis, hamstrings and gastrocnemius are the main muscles that must examined when considering patellofemoral pain.

- Inflexible tensor fascia latae moves posteriorly to the lateral femoral condyle during knee flexion, causing the patella to tilt and track laterally. This can be verified by the use of Ober's and Noble's tests. This lateral patella tracking produces patellofemoral pain. [8]
- If the vastus lateralis is asymmetrically stronger than the vastus medialis, the patella will tilt and track laterally during knee flexion, precipitating patellofemoral pain. [2,4,16]
- Inflexible hamstring muscles facilitate greater knee flexion, which acts adversely to the events during the gait cycle. Increased knee flexion warrants greater dorsi-flexion to clear the ground. [8,10,11,16]
- Inflexible gastrocnemius muscles inhibit the essential 10° of dorsi-flexion to clear the ground during the swing phase. This produces excessive sub-talar motion that increases internal tibial rotation, which facilitates a valgus force at the tibio-femoral joint. [8,11]

3. Special Non-Invasive Clinical Tests

Other special clinical tests that can be used to determine intrinsic risk of patella pain and injury include:

i. Quadriceps angle (Q-angle)
ii. A-angle
iii. Torsion angle
iv. Patellar orientation.

3.1. Quadriceps Angle

The quadriceps angle is a clinical measurement that quantifies the overall line of pull of the quadriceps muscles relative to the patellar tendon. The Q-angle can be measured according to the method described by Livingstone and Spaulding, with the subject lying supine on the plinth with feet in the neutral position. The anterior superior iliac spine (ASIS), the center of the patella and the tibial tuberosity are marked. The center of the goniometer is placed on the center of the patella (found by the intersecting width and length lines). The stationary arm of the goniometer is aligned with ASIS and the movable arm is aligned with the tibial tuberosity. A third vertical line that extends from the tibial tuberosity upwards along the femur enables the formation of an angle with the ASIS. The normative quadriceps angle for males is 10° and females is 15°. [7] The quadriceps angle is increased by lateral displacement of the tibial tuberosity, external tibial rotation, and increased torsion angle of the femur and the presence of coxa vara. Deviant quadriceps angles (greater than 15°) produce a valgus force at the tibio-femoral joint, which precipitates lateral tracking of the patella during flexion and pain. [17,19]

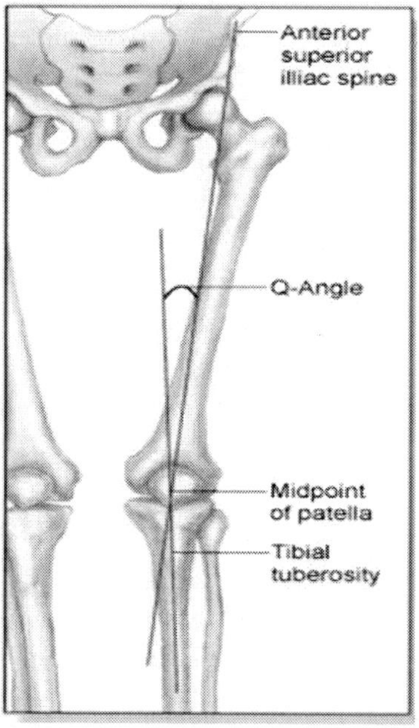

Figure 3. Visual representation of the landmarks of the quadriceps angle (www. Vesalius.com).

3.2. A-Angle

The A-angle measures the patellar orientation of the tibial tubercle. [8] A longitudinal line that bisects the patella is intersected by a line drawn from the tibial tubercle to the apex of the inferior pole of the patella. An A-angle greater than 35° is positively associated with patellofemoral pain in both men and women.

3.3. Torsion Angle

In adults, normal alignment places the femoral neck in a line that is 15° anterior to the line of femoral diaphysis.

Anteversion occurs when this angle of torsion is greater than 15°, the femur and tibia being medially rotated. Anteversion facilitates medial hip rotation, medial squinting patella and foot adduction, causing the person to walk with a toe-in gait appearance. Anteversion increases the presence of genu valgum, which increases the quadriceps angle. Increased quadriceps angles facilitate lateral tracking of the patella during flexion and/or extension of the tibia femoral joint. These lower limb misalignments increase the likelihood of PFPS.

Retroversion occurs when the angle of torsion is less than 15°, resulting in the lower limb being laterally rotated. Variations in the torsion angle alter the knee alignment and increase the risk of patellofemoral pain. Retroversion produces lateral hip rotation, frog-eyed (lateral squinting) patella and foot abduction, causing toe-gait. Femoral anteversion can be measured using Craig's test. [12]

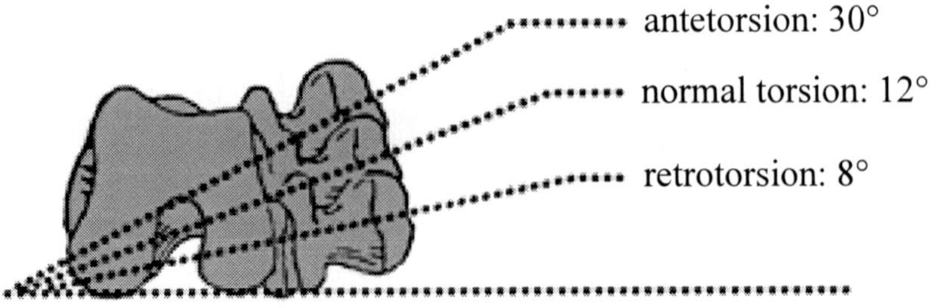

Figure 4. Variation in the femoral torsion angles.

3.4. Patellar Orientation

Patellar orientation is the positioning of the patella relative to the femoral trochlea and tibia. The assessment is conducted with the patient lying supine. The following four components must be assessed: glide, tilt, rotation and anteroposterior tilt.

- The *glide* component evaluates the lateral and/or medial deviation of the patella relative to the trochlea of the femur. Excessive gliding indicates the risk of patella mal-tracking. [5,8]
- The *tilt* component is determined by comparing the height of the medial and lateral patella borders. Difference in medial or lateral heights suggests a reduction of the impingement interval between the retro patellar surface and the femoral trochlear, which increases the risk of friction between the aforementioned bones during flexion and extension. [5,8]
- The *rotational* component evaluates the deviation of the longitudinal axis of the patella relative to the femur. The longitudinal axis is a line drawn from the superior to inferior poles of the patella, with the inferior pole being the point of reference. If the inferior pole is laterally deviated from the superior pole, this confirms external rotation of the patella. [8]
- The *anteroposterior* tilt component evaluates whether the surface of the patella is parallel to the longitudinal axis of the femur. The anteroposterior tilt is evaluated laterally to determine whether the longitudinal line drawn from the superior to inferior poles is parallel to the longitudinal axis of the femur. Anteroposterior tilt is confirmed when the inferior pole is posterior to the superior pole of the patellar. [8]

4. Consequences of Misalignment of Joint Along the Kinetic Chain

Misalignment of joints above and below the tibio-femoral joint influences the risk of knee injury and pain. In this brief section, the misalignment of the metatarsal joints and the lumbo-pelvic complex will be addressed.

- Knee pain is common among endurance runners, whose aetiology can be traced to pes planus, which can be attributed to a drop in navicular height due to increased laxity of the talonavicular, tibionavicular and dorsal cuboideonavicular ligaments. [21] This dropped navicular height propagates caudal displacement and internal rotation of the tibia, which stresses the medial patellar restraint. The medial patellar restraint comprises of the vastus medialis oblique, medial collateral ligament and anterior cruciate ligament. [4] Repetitive and prolonged stressing of the medial patellar restraint reduces its effectiveness against traction force of the lateral patellar restraint. This medial patellar restraint inefficiency produces lateral patella tracking, indicated by the abnormally larger quadriceps angle, which precipitates the onset of patellar femoral pain syndrome (PFPS). [21] Symptoms of PFPS are localized pain in and around the patellar, reduced range of motion, inflammation and crepitus. [8,11] Clinical identification of PFPS is a measurement of the quadriceps angle in excess of 10° and 15° for males and females, respectively. [7] This case study elaborates the adverse effects of misalignment up the kinetic chain, which are commonly referred to as serial distortion of the kinetic chain. [8]

- Athletes who have a lordotic posture have tight iliopsoas muscles and lengthened gluteal muscles. This altered force couple relationship between the iliopsoas and gluteal muscles affects the activation and subsequent force generation of these muscles. The tight iliopsoas muscle produces reciprocal inhibition, which allows the gluteal muscles to have a decreased neural drive, which adversely affects the person's hip extension. [8] If the gluteal muscles exert a weak hip extension moment, then the synergists of hip extension (hamstrings) become over-activated. Prolonged over-activation of the synergists leads to synergistic dominance. Synergistic dominance of the hamstrings will negatively impact their dynamic restraint capability to assist the ACL. Weakened and laxed ACL increases the intrinsic risk of ACL sprains and PFPS. [8]

REFERENCES

[1] Bahr, R. & Maehlum, S. (2004). Clinical guide to sport injuries. Champaign, IL: *Human Kinetics*

[2] Van der Worp, H., Van Ark, M., Roerink, S., Pepping, G., Van der Akker-Scheek, I., Zwerver, J. (2011). Risk factors for patellar tendinopathy: a systematic review of the literature. *British Journal of Sports Medicine*, 45: 446-52.

[3] Marieb, E. (2004). Human Anatomy and Physiology (7th edition). *Benjamin Cummings Publishing Company*

[4] Mansfield, P.J. & Neumann, D.A. (2012). Essential of Kinesiology for the Physical Therapist's Assistance. *Mosby: Elsevier.*

[5] Starke, C. & Ryan, F.L. (2001). Evaluation of Orthopaedic and Athletic Injuries (2nd edition). Philadelphia: USA

[6] Kendall, F.P., Mccreary, E.K., Provance, P.G., Rodgers, M.M. & Romani, W.A. (2005). Muscles: Testing and Function with Posture and Pain (5th edition), *Lippincott Williams & Wilkins,* Philadelphia, USA.

[7] Kent, M. (2005). Oxford Dictionary of Sports Science and Medicine. United Kingdom: *Oxford University Press.*

[8] Prentice WE. (2012). Rehabilitation Techniques for Sports Medicine and Athletic Training. Champaign, IL: *Human Kinetics.*

[9] Chomiak, J., Junge, A., Peterseon, L. (2000). Severe injuries in football players. Influencing factors. *American Journal of Sports Medicine*, 28: S58-68.

[10] Ekstrand, J. & Gillquist, J. (1983). Soccer injuries and their mechanisms: a prospective study. *Medicine and Science in Sport and Exercise,*15: 267-70.

[11] Brukner, P. & Khan, K. Clinical Sports Medicine (3rd edition). New York: *The McGraw Hill Company,* 2006.

[12] Houglum PA (2006). Therapeutic Exercises for Musculoskeletal Injuries. 3rd Ed. *Human Kinetics.*

[13] Twellaar, M., Verstappen, F.T., Huson, A. (1997). Physical characteristics as a risk factor for sport injuries: a four year prospective study. *International Journal of Sports Medicine,* 18: 66-71.

[14] Kaufman, K.R., Brodine, S.K., Shaffer, R.A. (1999). The effect of foot structure and range of motion on musculoskeletal overuse injuries. *American Journal of Sports Medicine,* 27: 585-93.

[15] Murphy, D.F., Connolly, D.A.J., Beynnon, B.D. (2003). Risk factors for lower extremity injury: a review of literature. *British Journal of Sport Medicine,* 37: 13-29.

[16] Witvrouw, E., Bellemans, J., Lysen, R. (2001). Intrinsic risk factors for developing patella tendinitis ian an athletic population. A two year prospective study. *American Journal of Sports Medicine,* 29: 190-5.

[17] Soderman, K. Alfredson, H. Pietila, T. (2001). Risk factors for leg injuries in female soccer players: a prospective investigation during one out door season. *Knee Surgery Sports Trauma,* 9: 313-21.

[18] Livingston, L.A. & Spaulding, S.J. (2002). Measuring of the quadriceps angle using standardized foot positions. *Journal of Athletic Training;* 37: 252-5.

[19] Shambaugh, J.P., Klein, A., Herbert, J.H. (1991). Structural measures as predictors of injury in basketball players. *Medicine and Science in Sport and Exercise,* 23: 522-7.

[20] Cowan, D.N., Jones, B.H., Frykman, P.N. (1996). Lower limb morphology and risk of overuse injury among male infantry recruits. *Medicine and Science in Sport and Exercise,* 28: 945-52.

[21] Ellapen, T.J., Chetty, L., Dorsamy, C., Abrahams, S., Desai, F.A., Narsigan, S. Van Heerden, H.J. (2011). Prevalence of triathlon musculoskeletal pain among tri-athletes in KZN, South Africa. *African Journal of Physical Health Education Recreation and Dance,* 17:112-23.

INDEX

A

accelerometers, 71
acetabulum, vii, 1, 2, 3, 5, 8, 10, 14, 20, 21, 22, 24, 26, 32, 33, 35, 37, 41, 48, 50
ACL, 138, 139, 140, 146
activity level, 27, 34, 35, 39
adaptations, xi, 123, 125, 126, 127, 128, 129, 134, 135
adduction, 9, 25, 144
adductor, 12, 139
adductor brevis, 139
adductor longus, 139
adolescents, x, 65, 103, 106, 132, 134
adulthood, 3
adults, 68, 144
adverse effects, 146
aesthetics, 66
aetiology, 145
age, 27, 34, 57, 58, 59, 60, 66, 99, 106, 110, 113, 115, 116, 117, 119, 120, 133
aggression, 53, 92
agility, 38
agonist, xi, 124, 127, 129
American Heart Association, 136
amplitude, 90
anatomy, 4, 22, 25, 32, 138
aneurysm, 58, 59
anger, 92
antagonist muscle strength, xi, 124
anterior cruciate, 138, 146
anti-inflammatories, 30
anti-inflammatory medications, 12
anxiety, 103, 104
aorta, 131
apex, 144
ARF, ix, 63, 64, 65, 66, 67, 68, 69, 72, 73, 74, 75, 76, 77, 80
Argentina, 108
arousal, 100
arteries, 58
artery, 33, 42, 58, 59
arthritis, viii, 1, 21, 31, 33, 42
arthroplasty, 49
arthroscopic-based procedures, viii, 2, 37
arthroscopy, 33, 34, 36, 38, 39, 40, 41, 42, 45, 46, 47, 48, 50
articular cartilage, 24, 49, 50
assessment, 13, 22, 25, 32, 36, 42, 43, 46, 57, 74, 80, 97, 98, 99, 135, 140, 145
assessment procedures, 97
asymptomatic, 6, 7, 9, 21, 22, 24, 29, 42, 43, 48
athletes, viii, ix, xi, 1, 2, 5, 7, 9, 12, 13, 22, 27, 28, 29, 32, 34, 36, 38, 39, 40, 42, 45, 46, 49, 52, 53, 56, 57, 58, 64, 79, 83, 87, 88, 90, 91, 94, 95, 96, 98, 100, 101, 103, 104, 123, 124, 125, 127, 128, 129, 130, 131, 132, 133, 134, 135, 148
athletic population, vii, 1, 22, 26, 29, 34, 36, 38, 147

athletic pubalgia, vii, 1, 9, 12, 42
attitudes, 65, 66, 67, 83
Austria, 100
autogenic training, 97
autopsy, 58, 59, 60
avascular necrosis, 12, 14, 37, 41
axial skeleton, 128

B

back pain, vii, 1, 138
basal ganglia, 57
behaviors, 91, 92
benefits, vii, xi, 28, 111, 119, 123, 124, 131, 132, 134, 138
biceps femoris, 139
biofeedback training, 97, 100
biomarkers, 24
biomechanical forces, ix, 87
biomechanics, 27, 28, 30, 49
bleeding, 77
blood, 33, 58, 59, 131, 136
blood pressure, 131
blood supply, 33
body composition, 133
body mass, vii, 45, 138
body mass index (BMI), 45
bone(s), xi, 3, 19, 21, 27, 32, 36, 55, 115, 123, 125, 127, 128, 131, 132, 133, 134, 136, 145
bone cells, 128
bone form, 3, 19, 27, 32, 128
bone growth, 128
bone marrow, 36
bone mass, 127, 128
bone mineral content, 125, 128
brain, viii, 51, 57, 59, 60, 65, 72, 102, 103, 129
brainstem, 57, 58, 59
breakdown, 6, 126
bursitis, vii, 1, 9, 22, 34

C

calcifications, 17, 20, 43
calcium, 128
CAM, 19
Cam lesions, vii, 1
capsule, 23
carotid arteries, 58
cartilage, viii, 1, 2, 3, 22, 24, 25, 30, 32, 33, 35, 36, 37, 39, 47, 50, 116, 125
case studies, 104, 146
cataract, 114
causal relationship, 27
causation, 7, 26
cbc, 61
central nervous system (CNS), viii, 51, 52, 53, 55, 60, 90
cerebral cortex, 57
cerebral edema, 55
cerebral hemisphere, 59
cerebrospinal fluid, 56
certification, 84
childhood, 3, 27, 48, 49
children, 44, 53, 132, 134
chronic diseases, 124
clinical assessment, 40
clinical examination, 38
clinical trials, 135
closure, 27, 135
clusters, 57
coaches, 67, 81, 133
coccyx, 13, 15
cognition, 100, 102
cognitive impairment, 69
coherence, 89
collagen, 127
collateral, 139
collisions, 53, 54
coma, 60
communication, 22, 95
communication skills, 95
community, 65, 67, 68, 77, 84
compartment syndrome, 37, 41
compensation, 79, 85
competition, 5, 22, 36, 52, 128

competitiveness, 132, 133
complex interactions, 99
compliance, ix, 64, 76, 77, 79, 133
complications, 33, 34, 36, 38, 40, 46, 48, 130
composition, 72, 73
compression, 140
concussion, viii, ix, 52, 53, 55, 60, 63, 64, 65, 66, 67, 70, 71, 72, 73, 74, 75, 76, 77, 78, 79, 80, 81, 82, 84
conditioning, xi, 123, 125, 132, 133, 134
congenital dysplasia, 50
connective tissue, xi, 123, 125, 127, 134, 136
consciousness, 53, 55, 58, 60
construction, 66, 72, 75
contact sport, viii, x, 51, 57, 69, 105
contour, 24, 46
control group, 27, 96, 97
controlled trials, ix, 63, 76, 79, 98
contusion, 12, 55
convention, 30
coping strategies, 96
coronary heart disease, vii, 138
cortex, 57
counseling, 36
coxa plana, 49
crepitus, 146
cross-sectional study, 47, 76, 121
crystals, 128
CT scan, 13, 25, 26, 41, 42, 45, 46
cyst, 14, 31

D

daily living, 30
dancers, 7, 28, 41, 43, 95, 97, 103
data collection, 99
debridement, 33, 35, 36, 44
deceleration forces, viii, 51, 52
defects, 5, 23, 36, 43, 47
deficiency, 19, 32, 76
deficit, 54
deformation, 70
degenerative joint disease, 3
dental injuries, 114, 121
depth, 3, 17, 24, 32, 38, 57
detection, 21, 22, 23, 24, 26
deviation, 20, 140, 145
diabetes, vii, 138
dialysis, 114
diaphysis, 144
differential diagnosis, 11
disability, 5, 6, 26, 30
discomfort, ix, 25, 42, 63, 68, 69, 80, 117
diseases, vii, 90, 138
dislocation, 33, 34, 39, 41, 45, 46, 48, 49, 50, 54
displacement, 143, 146
distress, 92
distribution, 57, 111, 112
dominance, 146
dyslipidemia, 124
dysplasia, viii, 2, 5, 9, 12, 14, 21, 46

E

edema, 55
education, 28, 32, 38, 60, 81
emergency, x, 105, 109, 111, 112, 115, 119
emotion regulation, 92
emotional state, 102
encephalopathy, 52, 57
endurance, 124, 125, 130, 135, 145
energy, ix, 56, 65, 83, 87
energy transfer, ix, 87
enforcement, 81
entrapment, 3
environmental conditions, vii, 138
epidemic, 52
epidemiologic, 49
epidemiology, 84
epidural hematoma, 52, 60
epiphyses, 3
epiphysis, viii, 2, 48, 50
equipment, vii, x, 28, 52, 64, 76, 81, 83, 84, 105, 106, 109, 110, 111, 112, 113, 116, 118, 119, 120, 121, 138
ethylene, 73
etiology, 22, 40, 41

Europe, 108
event-related potential, 90
everyday life, 96
evidence, ix, x, xi, 6, 7, 21, 22, 24, 27, 28, 29, 30, 31, 32, 55, 57, 58, 64, 76, 79, 80, 88, 90, 97, 124, 128, 132, 133, 136
evoked potential, 102
evolution, 46
execution, xi, 124
exercise, 31, 101, 126, 127, 128, 130, 131, 132, 133, 135, 136, 139
exertion, 131
experimental design, 97
exposure, 79, 132
extensor, 135
extravasation, 39

F

facial injuries, x, 106, 112, 114, 119
fat, 24, 133
fears, 52, 92
female rat, 113
femoroacetabular impingement (FAI), vii, 1, 2, 3, 5, 6, 7, 8, 9, 11, 12, 13, 14, 17, 19, 20, 21, 22, 24, 25, 26, 28, 29, 30, 32, 33, 34, 37, 38, 39, 40, 41, 42, 43, 44, 45, 46, 47, 48, 49, 50
femur, vii, 1, 2, 3, 5, 7, 10, 22, 24, 32, 41, 48, 138, 139, 140, 143, 144, 145
fibers, 9, 127
fibrin, 36, 49
field sports, x, 105, 106
fitness, xi, 124, 131, 135
fixation, 33, 34, 43
flex, 139
flexibility, 90, 92
flexor, 127
fluid, 39
foams, 75
football, ix, 7, 22, 28, 43, 44, 45, 48, 63, 64, 68, 76, 81, 82, 83, 84, 85, 88, 93, 94, 100, 111, 116, 122, 147
football injuries, 94, 100
football positions, 28
force, 2, 3, 10, 56, 65, 70, 71, 126, 127, 129, 134, 135, 139, 140, 142, 143, 146
formation, 14, 17, 28, 31, 38, 143
foundations, 101
fractures, x, 5, 20, 41, 54, 77, 78, 106, 111, 114, 115, 122, 128, 131, 134
friction, 145
funding, 61
fusion, 102

G

gadolinium, 22, 23
gait, 9, 29, 142, 144
gastrocnemius, 142
gel, 41, 42
general anaesthesia, 115, 119
genu recurvatum, xii, 137, 140
genu valgum, xii, 137, 140, 141, 144
genu varum, xii, 137, 141
geometry, 47
Germany, 49
glucocorticoids, 90, 91
gluteus maximus, 31, 139
goal-setting, 96, 97
gracilis, 139
growth, 27, 48, 99, 125, 126, 132
guidelines, 26, 28, 131
gymnasts, 94, 96, 102

H

hamstring, 31, 90, 99, 142
hand trauma, x, 106
handguards, x, 105, 106, 109, 118
head injuries, ix, x, 53, 64, 65, 74, 75, 76, 77, 78, 79, 80, 81, 83, 84, 105, 106, 110, 112, 115, 119, 121
head injury, ix, x, 63, 64, 65, 69, 70, 73, 74, 76, 77, 78, 79, 80, 81, 85, 106, 110, 118, 119, 120
head to head contact, ix, 63, 72, 80
head trauma, viii, x, 52, 53, 55, 57, 58, 60, 106, 112

headache, 55, 58
headgear, ix, 63, 64, 65, 66, 67, 68, 69, 70, 71, 72, 73, 74, 75, 76, 77, 78, 79, 80, 81, 82, 83, 84, 85, 119
healing, 126
health, vii, 24, 28, 52, 60, 124, 127, 131, 132, 133, 134, 135, 138
health care, 60
health promotion, 28
health risks, 131
height, 74, 75, 106, 109, 140, 145
helmets, x, 60, 64, 82, 105, 106, 109, 111, 113, 114, 116, 117, 118, 119, 120, 121
hematoma, 55
hemorrhage, 52, 59, 60
herniated nucleus pulposus, 12
heterogeneity, 36
high school, 53, 65, 67, 83
Highlands, 121
hip arthroplasty, 22, 33, 49
hip joint, vii, 1, 2, 9, 20, 22, 25, 32, 42, 43
Hong Kong, 41
hormones, 90, 102
human cognition, 102
hyper-extension, xii, 137
hypertension, 59
hypertrophy, 125, 126, 127, 129
hypokinetic diseases, vii, 138

I

iatrogenic, 33, 36, 45
identification, 22, 26, 30, 34, 96, 120, 146
idiopathic, 5, 49
idiosyncratic, 89, 98
iliac crest, 12
iliopsoas, 12, 31, 40, 146
imagery, 93, 97
images, 13, 20, 21, 22, 23, 24, 25
imaging modalities, viii, 2
imbalances, xi, 124
impact energy, 65, 73, 74, 75
improvements, xi, 123, 128, 129
impulsive, 92
incidence, viii, x, xi, 7, 9, 29, 34, 41, 42, 51, 52, 53, 60, 64, 65, 69, 70, 78, 79, 80, 82, 88, 93, 95, 106, 121, 123, 130, 133
independent variable, 99
individualization, 38
individuals, xi, 3, 5, 6, 9, 21, 24, 30, 32, 36, 43, 54, 57, 90, 124, 126, 130, 131, 133
ineffectiveness, 133
inefficiency, 146
infarction, 59
inflammation, 12, 146
inguinal, 12
inhibition, 26, 38, 80, 146
injury prevention, 85, 92, 93, 95, 96, 100, 104, 125, 127, 129, 132, 133, 135
inoculation, 96
integrity, 127, 133
internal fixation, 41, 44, 119
intervention, 29, 30, 32, 38, 40, 76, 79, 93, 94, 96, 97, 98, 99, 100, 101, 103, 104
intervention strategies, 93
intravenously, 23
ipsilateral, 13
Ireland, 105, 108, 110, 113, 122
isolation, 3, 93

J

joints, 127, 138, 145
Jordan, 83
jumping, 9, 126, 128

K

Kendall protocol, xii, 137
knee injury, xii, 136, 137, 145
knees, xii, 13, 137, 140

L

laboratory studies, 69, 72
labrum, viii, 1, 3, 9, 20, 22, 23, 25, 32, 33, 35, 36, 43, 44, 49
laceration, 78, 114, 115

latency, 58
lateral collateral, 139
lateral meniscus, 140
lead, 3, 7, 90, 91
legislation, 116
legs, 29
lesions, vii, 1, 6, 19, 21, 24, 26, 35, 49, 50, 103
ligament, 45, 125, 131, 140, 146
light, 28, 76, 92
linear model, 99
locus, 89
loss of consciousness, 53, 55
lumbar spine, 12

M

magnesium, 71, 73, 74, 75
magnetic resonance imaging (MRI), 13, 22, 24, 39, 40, 41, 43, 44, 47, 48, 49
magnitude, 22, 74, 128
management, vii, viii, 2, 12, 30, 32, 33, 35, 36, 37, 38, 39, 40, 46, 48, 81, 89, 93, 94, 95, 96, 97, 100, 102, 103
mandible, 119
manipulation, 115
martial art, 66, 70
mass, vii, 70, 72, 126, 127, 128, 133, 138
mastoid, 59
materials, 75, 80, 102
matrix, 127, 128
measurement, 17, 24, 39, 41, 47, 143, 146
media, viii, 52, 53, 59, 64
medial collateral, 138, 146
medial meniscus, 140
medical, viii, 2, 56, 67, 109, 132
medicine, xii, 61, 64, 134, 137
memory, 76, 92
Mercury, 61
meta-analysis, 48
metabolism, 126
metatarsal, 145
military, 6, 56
Missouri, 134
modelling, 99, 128
models, 99
moderating factors, 91
moisture, 66
molecules, 128
mood states, 103
morbidity, ix, 87
morphology, 2, 3, 5, 6, 7, 9, 20, 22, 24, 25, 27, 28, 29, 30, 32, 38, 39, 42, 45, 46, 129, 148
motivation, 69, 89, 99
motor skills, 133
mouthguard, 77
mouthguards, x, 105, 109
multidimensional, 13
muscle relaxation, 93
muscle strain, 115
muscle strength, vii, xi, 123, 124, 126, 127, 128, 136, 138
muscles, xi, 30, 123, 126, 127, 129, 130, 131, 135, 139, 140, 142, 143, 146
muscular injuries, x, 106, 110
musculoskeletal, xi, 30, 90, 123, 124, 125, 126, 129, 130, 134, 147, 148
musculoskeletal injuries, xi, 123, 124, 125, 126, 129, 130
musculoskeletal system, 125

N

National Survey, 61
neck injury, 82
negative reinforcement, 99
nerve, 37, 43, 54
nervous system, 61, 129
neurofibrillary tangles, 57
neuroimaging, 55
neuropraxia, 33, 37
neurosurgery, 61, 62
neutral, 13, 54, 81, 143
New Zealand, 82, 85, 96, 108
North America, 61
novelty seeking, 92
NSAIDs, 30
nuclei, 20
nutrition, 96

O

obesity, 27
organ, ix, 87
organizational stress, 101
organs, 127
ossicles, 42
ossification, 33, 34, 45
osteoarthritis, 5, 6, 12, 14, 26, 27, 29, 30, 33, 39, 40, 41, 46, 49, 136
osteoporosis, vii, 128, 138
osteotomy, 32, 33, 34, 45, 47, 48, 50
outcome relationship, 91

P

pain, vii, xii, 1, 2, 5, 6, 7, 8, 9, 10, 11, 12, 21, 22, 23, 26, 27, 30, 31, 32, 33, 34, 38, 39, 43, 44, 46, 48, 56, 95, 102, 137, 140, 142, 143, 144, 145, 148
pain management, 30
palpation, 9
parallel, 13, 15, 17, 24, 29, 145
paralysis, viii, 52, 53
participants, 66, 67, 68, 69, 76, 77, 78, 80, 91, 109
patella, xii, 137, 138, 140, 141, 142, 143, 144, 145, 146, 147
patellar tendon, 140, 143
patho-anatomic relationships, viii, 2
pathogenesis, 38, 92
pathology, vii, 1, 2, 3, 8, 9, 10, 12, 22, 24, 28, 29, 32, 35, 36, 55, 57
pectineus, 139
pelvis, 6, 9, 12, 13, 20, 43
penalties, 52, 81
performers, 101
periosteum, 128
permeability, 56
personality factors, 89
personality research, 101
personality traits, 88
Perthes disease, viii, 2, 45
phalanges, 115
phalanx, 114, 115
Philadelphia, 147
phosphate, 128
physical activity, vii, xi, 3, 46, 123, 127, 130, 134, 138
physical therapist, 38
physical therapy, 30, 38
physicians, 54, 56
physiological health, vii, 138
pilot study, 83, 84, 100, 121
Pincer lesions, vii, 1
placebo, 96
playing, vii, 32, 53, 57, 58, 64, 66, 74, 79, 82, 91, 103, 109, 111, 112, 115, 117, 118, 119, 120, 121, 138
policy, 119
polyether, 75
polyurethane, 75
population, vii, 1, 6, 7, 9, 21, 22, 26, 29, 34, 36, 38, 44, 147
posterior cruciate, 138
preservation, 33, 36, 98
prevention, vii, 26, 28, 29, 30, 32, 38, 40, 68, 82, 84, 94, 98, 99, 101, 102, 111, 119, 121, 124, 125, 128, 129, 130, 131, 132, 133
prognosis, 45
prophylactic, 27
prophylaxis, 26
protection, x, xi, 66, 68, 71, 74, 75, 91, 106, 112, 116, 118, 119, 120, 121, 123, 126, 127
protective factors, 85
psychologist, 94
psychology, 90, 92, 103, 104
psychosocial factors, 88, 89, 96, 102
pubis, 9, 12, 13, 22

Q

quadriceps, xii, 31, 137, 139, 143, 144, 146, 148

R

Rab, 5, 47
radius, 19, 21, 24
Ramadan, 39
reaction time, 90, 104
reactivity, 90, 93, 98
reconstruction, 35, 36, 39, 42, 84
recovery, xi, 27, 37, 69, 82, 124, 126
recreation, 122
recreational, xi, 104, 123, 124, 125, 131
rectus femoris, 20, 47, 139
regulations, 75, 81, 119, 121
rehabilitation, xi, 30, 38, 124
rehabilitation program, 38
relaxation, 95, 96, 97
reliability, 9, 13, 21, 40
relief, 23, 33
remodelling, 129
repair, 12, 35, 36, 47, 49, 114
repetitions, 125
requirements, 66, 110, 130, 134
researchers, ix, 64, 76, 88, 96, 118
resection, 32, 33, 36, 48
resilience, 66
resistance, xi, 9, 28, 123, 124, 125, 126, 127, 128, 129, 130, 131, 132, 133, 134, 135, 136, 139
resistance exercises, xi, 123
resistance training, xi, 123, 124, 125, 126, 127, 128, 129, 130, 131, 132, 133, 134, 135, 136
resolution, 22
resources, 89, 92, 104
response, 20, 22, 23, 48, 89, 90, 92, 128, 129
restoration, 38
rhythm, 102
risk, vii, viii, xi, xii, 1, 6, 17, 23, 26, 27, 28, 29, 41, 45, 46, 49, 52, 53, 58, 66, 69, 70, 71, 74, 76, 77, 78, 79, 80, 82, 84, 85, 90, 91, 92, 96, 100, 101, 102, 103, 104, 109, 119, 120, 123, 124, 125, 126, 128, 129, 130, 131, 132, 136, 137, 138, 139, 142, 144, 145, 146, 147, 148
risk factors, vii, xii, 26, 82, 101, 131, 136, 137, 138, 139, 147
risk profile, 90
risk-taking, 91, 92, 103
roots, 54
rugby, ix, 63, 64, 65, 66, 68, 69, 72, 73, 74, 75, 76, 79, 80, 81, 82, 83, 84, 85, 95, 96, 116
rules, 81, 84, 119, 132

S

safety, 53, 116, 117, 132
scar tissue, 38
sclerosis, 12, 14, 31
search terms, viii, 52, 53, 65
security, 79, 117
self-confidence, 94, 95, 96
self-control, 95, 100
self-reports, 98
semimembranosus, 139
sensation, 56
sensitivity, 9, 24, 91
shape, 23, 27
shear, 2, 3, 10
shinguards, x, 105, 109
shoot, 52
signs, viii, 2, 6, 12, 20, 21, 29, 57
skeletal alignment, vii, 138
skeletal muscle, 124, 126, 134
skills training, 81, 95, 97
skin, 116
skull fracture, 64, 65, 66
slipped capital femoral epiphysis, 26, 40, 42, 43, 45, 47
soccer, ix, 7, 22, 28, 29, 42, 43, 44, 63, 64, 65, 66, 69, 70, 71, 72, 74, 76, 80, 81, 83, 84, 93, 95, 96, 97, 99, 101, 103, 147
social stress, 92, 103
social support, 89, 91, 96, 103
social support network, 89
South Africa, 29, 104, 108, 123, 137, 148
Spain, 87
Spaulding technique, xii, 138
specifications, 81

spinal cord, viii, 51, 52, 53, 54, 56, 60
spinal cord injury, viii, 52, 54, 60
spinal stenosis, 55
spine, x, 16, 20, 43, 54, 106, 110, 143
splinting, 115
spondylolisthesis, 12
sport participation, vii, 138
sport practitioner, ix, 87
sports performance, xi, 123, 124
sprains, 54, 116, 131, 140, 146
stability, 44, 132
stabilization, 35
state(s), 50, 90, 92, 100
steel, 72, 74, 75
stenosis, 56
stereotyping, 100
stimulation, 36
stimulus, 129
strength training, 90, 124, 125, 128, 129, 132, 134, 135, 136
stress, ix, 12, 13, 20, 22, 45, 87, 88, 89, 90, 91, 92, 93, 94, 95, 96, 97, 98, 99, 100, 102, 103, 104, 134, 139, 140
stress fracture, 12, 13, 20, 22, 45, 134
stress response, x, 87, 88, 89, 91, 102
stress test, 140
stressful events, 89
stressful life events, 88
stressors, 89, 96, 100, 104
stretching, 30, 90
structure, 128, 147
stupor, 58
subarachnoid hemorrhage, 52, 55, 59, 60
subdural hematoma, 52, 55, 60
subluxation, 12, 45, 50
substance abuse, 57
Sun, 59, 62, 82
supervision, xi, 124
surgical intervention, 14, 32
Sweden, 101, 102
swelling, 55, 56
symmetry, 13, 15
symptoms, 5, 6, 8, 9, 10, 12, 13, 17, 22, 29, 30, 42, 55, 56, 79
syndrome, viii, 11, 47, 52, 55, 60, 146

T

target populations, 134
targeted resistance-based approach, xi, 124
tau, 57
teams, 59, 67, 77, 78, 79, 81, 95, 97
techniques, xii, 29, 30, 33, 36, 37, 93, 95, 99, 132, 137
technology, 80, 99, 102
teeth, x, 106, 110
tendinitis, 47, 147
tendon, 12, 40, 125, 127, 131, 140
tendons, 125
tension, 53, 90, 93, 102, 142
tensor fascia lata, 139, 142
testing, xi, 70, 72, 74, 93, 97, 99, 124
theoretical approaches, 101
therapist, 30
therapy, 32
three-dimensional reconstruction, 13
tibia, 138, 139, 140, 141, 144, 145, 146
tibio-femoral alignment, xii, 137
tibio-femoral joint, xii, 137, 138, 139, 142, 143, 145
tissue, ix, xi, xii, 22, 35, 47, 56, 65, 84, 87, 114, 115, 123, 126, 127, 128, 137
torsion, xii, 137, 143, 144
trade-off, 66
training, x, xi, 28, 90, 93, 94, 95, 96, 97, 104, 105, 109, 113, 115, 123, 124, 125, 126, 127, 128, 129, 130, 131, 132, 133, 134, 135, 136
training programs, xi, 93, 123, 124, 128, 130, 131, 132, 135, 136
trait anxiety, 89
translation, 31, 139
trauma, x, 20, 55, 57, 58, 106, 112, 121, 126
traumatic brain injury, 57, 81, 85
treatment, vii, 1, 13, 26, 29, 30, 31, 32, 33, 34, 38, 39, 40, 41, 43, 45, 46, 48, 49, 50, 96, 97, 98
trial, ix, 32, 64, 67, 69, 76, 78, 84, 103, 118
triggers, 89
trochanter, 8, 9, 12, 13, 33, 34, 39
trochanteric bursitis, vii, 1, 9